MRCP Part 2

Best of Five Illustrated
Questions and Answers

Commissioning Editor: Ellen Green, Pauline Graham
Project Development Manager: Clive Hewat
Project Manager: Andrew Palfreyman
Designer: Erik Bigland

MRCP Part 2

Data Interpretation Questions and Answers

Huw Beynon BSc MD FRCP

Consultant Physician
Department of Rheumatology
Royal Free Hospital
London

Luke Gompels MA MRCP

Specialist Registrar Rheumatology and General Internal Medicine
Department of Rheumatology
Hammersmith Hospital
London

Rapti Mediwake MRCP

Consultant Rheumatologist and General Physician
Department Rheumatology
Barner Hospital
Hertfordshire

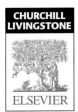

CHURCHILL
LIVINGSTONE

ELSEVIER

Edinburgh   London   New York   Oxford   Philadelphia   St Louis   Sydney   Toronto   2008

CHURCHILL
LIVINGSTONE
ELSEVIER

First edition 1991
Second edition 1998
Third edition 2008

ISBN: 9780443073304

British Library Cataloguing in Publication Data
A catalogue record for this book is available from the British Library

Library of Congress Cataloging in Publication Data
A catalog record for this book is available from the Library of Congress

Note
Medical knowledge is constantly changing. Standard safety precautions must be followed, but as new research and clinical experience broaden our knowledge, changes in treatment and drug therapy may become necessary or appropriate. Readers are advised to check the most current product information provided by the manufacturer of each drug to be administered to verify the recommended dose, the method and duration of administration, and contraindications. It is the responsibility of the practitioner, relying on experience and knowledge of the patient, to determine dosages and the best treatment for each individual patient. Neither the Publisher nor the authors assumes any liability for any injury and/or damage to persons or property arising from this publication.

The Publisher

ELSEVIER   your source for books,
            journals and multimedia
            in the health sciences
www.elsevierhealth.com

Working together to grow
libraries in developing countries
www.elsevier.com | www.bookaid.org | www.sabre.org

ELSEVIER   BOOK AID   Sabre Foundation
           International

The
publisher's
policy is to use
paper manufactured
from sustainable forests

Printed in Holland

This book has been prepared in the format of the MRCP examination – selecting a best answer from five. Questions and answers have been meticulously prepared to be both challenging and also to enable the examinee to gain a thorough understanding of both the clinical cases and other key disorders that the question stems raise – ensuring a broad range of related questions can be confidently answered.

Many of the cases here are based on real patient problems. It has been the authors' experience that the stimulation and satisfaction of working through these cases extends not only to passing the Membership but also to improving day-to-day clinical practice – we hope that you find the same.

We gratefully acknowledge the contributions of Professor JB van den Bogaerde and Professor KA Davies who were involved in previous editions of this book.

HLC Beynon
LL Gompels
R Mediwake
2007

Questions

A 40-year-old male has just been transferred from another hospital. He is known to have acute lymphoblastic leukaemia and to have undergone chemotherapy following which he developed a prolonged pyrexial illness requiring intravenous treatment. No other details are currently available. He is tired, listless and nauseous. He is normotensive. The clinical examination is otherwise unremarkable and his urine dip is negative.

The lab phones with the following results:

Sodium	137 mmol/L
Potassium	2.4 mmol/L
Urea	5.0 mmol/L
Bicarbonate	18 mmol/L
Chloride	110 mmol/L

What is the most likely diagnosis?

1. Recurrent vomiting
2. Bartter's syndrome
3. Addisonian crisis
4. Acquired renal tubular acidosis
5. Diabetic ketoacidosis

Question 02

An 80-year-old female is admitted from her warden-controlled flat having been found drowsy and unable to answer the door. There had been a history of previous similar episodes where she had made a good recovery with resuscitation at the emergency department.

On examination she is drowsy and flushed. Her temperature is 36.8°C, pulse 120/min, respiratory rate 18/min and blood pressure 160/80 mmHg. The remainder of her examination is unremarkable. Oxygen saturations by pulse oximetry are 99%.

A blood gas sample taken on air shows the following:

pH	7.3
pO_2	10.5 kPa
pCo_2	3.8 kPa
Bicarbonate	23 mmol/L
O_2 saturation	83%

What is the most likely cause for these results?

1. Type 2 respiratory failure
2. Carbon monoxide poisoning
3. Venous blood gas sample
4. Type 1 respiratory failure
5. Pulmonary embolism

Answer to Question 02 *is on page 182*

A 15-year-old female presents with a 2-month history of fatigue. She commenced her periods 18 months previously and these have recently become heavy. On three occasions in the past her mother has commented that she 'looks yellow'. Her father, who no longer lives at home, was diagnosed in his youth as having recurrent anaemia. She has no siblings and is not on medication. On examination she is pale and abdominal examination reveals 2-cm splenomegaly.

INVESTIGATIONS

Hb	6.6 g/dL
WBC	8.4×10^9/L
Platelets	385×10^9/L
Reticulocytosis	10%
Direct Coombs' test	negative
Sodium	141 mmol/L
Potassium	4.9 mmol/L
Urea	4.3 mmol/L
Bilirubin	38 μmol/L
Aspartate transaminase	69 iu/L
Alkaline phosphatase	119 iu/L
Haptoglobins	not detected
Urinary haemosiderin	absent

a) What is the likely diagnosis?
   1. Sickle cell anaemia
   2. Hereditary spherocytosis
   3. Thalassemia trait
   4. Gilbert's syndrome
   5. Systemic lupus erythematosus

b) The next most appropriate test would be:
   1. Haemoglobin electrophoresis
   2. Ultrasound abdomen
   3. Anti-nuclear antibodies
   4. Blood film
   5. Bone marrow aspirate and trephine

You are performing a medical outreach clinic and are asked to see a 31-year-old staff nurse who presents with tiredness and symptoms of numbness and tingling affecting all fingers of the right hand. The pain is intermittent but is most troublesome in the mornings. She has noticed a facial rash associated with localized hyperpigmentation.

General examination is unremarkable, with blood pressure of 105/70 mmHg and a pulse of 76/min. Axial and appendicular skeletal examination is normal. Tinel's sign is positive on the right side.

The available investigations show the following:

Sodium	132 mmol/L
Potassium	4.2 mmol/L
Urea	3.2 mmol/L
Creatinine	64 µmol/L

ALP 212 iu/L, AST 40 iu/L, Albumin 33 g/L, total protein 66 g/L, Hb 10.5 g/dL, normochromic normocytic; WCC 11.1 × 10^9/L, platelets 169 × 10^9/L. Complement levels: C3 120% of normal, C4 118% of normal human pool, CH50 17%.

a) Which of the following tests is most appropriate?
   1. Anti-mitochondrial and smooth muscle antibodies
   2. Liver biopsy
   3. Anti-nuclear antibody
   4. Ultrasound liver
   5. Urinalysis and βHCG levels

b) What is the most likely cause of the numbness in her right hand?
   1. Cervical myelopathy
   2. Peripheral neuropathy
   3. Carpal tunnel syndrome
   4. Ulnar nerve compression
   5. Multiple sclerosis

Answer to Question 04 *is on page 184*

A 45-year-old male has a long history of Reiter's disease. He attends casualty with a week's history of nausea and dizziness, diarrhoea and abdominal pain. Recurrent hip problems have resulted in him being scheduled to have a hip replacement in one week. He was taking leflunomide and prednisolone but he was requested to stop all medication prior to surgery other then diclofenac for pain relief.

On examination he is apyrexial and clinically dehydrated with dry mucous membranes. Lying blood pressure is 130/80 mmHg and standing blood pressure is 90/50 mmHg. His pulse rate is 100/min regular and heart sounds are normal. General examination is unremarkable aside from some mild epigastric tenderness.

INVESTIGATIONS

Hb	14.5 g/dL
WCC	8.78×10^9/L
Platelets	450×10^9/L
CRP	5 mg/L
Sodium	130 mmol/L
Potassuim	4.4 mmol/L
Urea	7.0 mmol/L
Creatinine	95 mmol/L

a) What is the most likely diagnosis?
  1. Acute peptic ulceration
  2. Infective endocarditis
  3. Hypoadrenalism
  4. Septic arthritis
  5. Urinary tract infection

b) What further test will help you with the diagnosis?
  1. Oesophagogastroduodenoscopy
  2. Transoesophagal echocardiogram
  3. Short synacthen test
  4. Urine microscopy
  5. Isotope bone scan

Answer to Question 05 *is on page 185*

A 30-year-old male presents with diffuse colicky abdominal pains and night sweats. He also has had a non-productive cough, anorexia and fevers up to 39°C accompanied by rigors and chills. After being prescribed antibiotics he felt well for 3 days but symptoms then recurred and were accompanied by a dull frontal headache, muscle pains and severe fatigue. He had not undertaken any foreign travel apart from a holiday visiting his grandparents in Kenya 1 month before. He had obtained malaria prophylaxis before leaving the UK.

On examination his temperature is 39.8°C, pulse 110/min, blood pressure 110/60 mmHg and respiratory rate 20/min. He is lethargic and belligerent when disturbed. There are no other signs of meningism. He has clear lung fields and a soft pansystolic murmur at the apex on cardiorespiratory examination. There is diffuse abdominal tenderness predominantly in the upper quadrants but no guarding or rebound. Neurological examination reveals no focal signs.

INVESTIGATIONS

Haematology

Hb 8.5 g/dL, MCV 87 fL, MCHC 30 pg, WBC 7×10^9/L – 62% neutrophils, platelets 118×10^9/L, ESR 80 mm in the first hour

Biochemistry

Glucose 6.2 mmol/L, sodium 130 mmol/L, potassium 4.0 mmol/L, bicarbonate 20 mmol/L, urea 30 mmol/L, creatinine 495 μmol/L

Bilirubin 12 μmol/L, alkaline phosphatase 50 iu/L, aspartate aminotransferase 70 iu/L, Lactate dehydrogenase 495 iu/L, amylase 60 iu/L, creatinine kinase 50 iu/L, albumin 28 g/L, total protein 65 g/L, calcium 1.7 mmol/L, phosphate 1.19 mmol/L

Miscellaneous

Urine dipstick tests: blood +, protein +++
Urine microscopy: several granular and hyaline casts seen per high power field
Chest and abdominal X-rays-normal
CT Head-normal

What is the most likely diagnosis?

1. Infective endocarditis
2. Falciparum malaria
3. Atypical pneumonia
4. Cerebral abscess
5. Cerebral systemic lupus erythematosus

Answer to Question 06 *is on page 186*

A 35-year-old female is admitted to casualty with status epilepticus. The convulsion is terminated with diazepam. On recovering consciousness she gives a history of severe abdominal pain and vomiting and admits to having had two previous fits. She has noted progressive weakness in her right arm and is unable to grip a tennis racquet properly. On examination she looks well, and is apyrexial with a regular pulse and blood pressure. There are no localizing signs in the abdomen. Neurologically there is a right radial nerve palsy – the rest of the examination is unremarkable.

INVESTIGATIONS

Sodium	123 mmol/L
Potassium	4.0 mmol/L
Urea	4 mmol/L
Bilirubin	35 µmol/L
Aspartate transaminase	42 iu/L

a) Suggest a unifying diagnosis:
  1. Mycoplasma pneumonia
  2. Systemic lupus erythematosus
  3. Acute intermittent porphyria
  4. Intracranial mass
  5. Campylobacter gastroenteritis

b) How would you confirm this diagnosis?
  1. Mycoplasma serology
  2. ANA
  3. CT head
  4. Urine-δ-aminolaevulinic acid
  5. Stool culture

A patient is HBsAg +, HepBeAg (–) and anti-HepBe (+). He has a HBV DNA of $<10^5$ copies/mL. Recent ALT/AST levels have been persistently normal.

What is his clinical status?

1. Chronic hepatitis B
2. Inactive carrier
3. Resolved hepatitis B
4. Acute hepatitis B
5. Recently immunized

Answer to Question 08 *is on page 189*

A 42-year-old bus driver is referred with a rash presumed to be second-ary to amoxicillin. He had presented to his GP 5 days before with a 6-day history of anorexia, fever and headache, and a 3-day history of dry cough and mild dyspnoea. He smokes 10 cigarettes per day. His past history is unremarkable. He had been commenced on amoxicillin 500 mg 8-hourly. On admission he was fully alert; his examination findings were: tempera-ture 39°C, pulse 90/min, blood pressure 110/60 mmHg. There was good air entry generally with no wheeze, but several fine crepitations could be heard in the right base. He had a fine maculopapular rash over his trunk and arms; several target lesions were noted. General examination was otherwise unremarkable. His amoxicillin was stopped and he was observed overnight. The following day he complains of generalized myalgia and dull central chest pain.

INVESTIGATIONS

Hb	13 g/dL
WBC	10×10^9/L
Sodium	142 mmol/L
Potassium	4.4 mmol/L
Urea	9 mmol/L
Creatinine	90 µmol/L
ESR	70 mm in the first hour
Aspartate transaminase	90 iu/L
Alkaline phosphatase	150 iu/L
Bilirubin	12 µmol/L
Blood and sputum culture	negative
Cold agglutinins	positive
Chest X-ray	patchy consolidation right base
Blood gases	PO_2 8.9 kPa, pCO_2 4.5 kPa
ECG	sinus tachycardia, widespread T-wave flattening and inversion

Echocardiography showed normal valves and chambers. Contraction of the left ventricle was reduced.

a) Suggest the most likely diagnosis:
1. Wegener's granulomatosis
2. *Mycoplasma pneumoniae*
3. Systemic lupus erythematosus
4. Chlamydia pneumonia
5. Coxsackie virus infection

Question continued overpage

b) What treatment would you give?
   1. High dose steroids
   2. Ganciclovir
   3. Intravenous ceftriaxzone
   4. Erythromycin
   5. Cyclophosphamide

Answer to Question 09 *is on page 191*

A 55-year-old male is admitted for investigation of recurrent peptic ulceration. His problems first started at 43 years of age when he was resident in India and was admitted for emergency surgery to repair a perforated peptic ulcer. Three years later he underwent a partial gastrectomy for recurrent peptic ulceration. Since that time he has been persistently troubled by abdominal pain which is worse at night, and diarrhoea with 4 loose motions a day. His current medication is ranitidine 150 mg 12-hourly, together with liberal doses of antacids.

INVESTIGATIONS

Hb	10 g/dL
MCV	76 fL
MCH	26 pg
MCHC	30 g/dL
Urea and electrolytes	normal
Liver function tests	normal
Fasting serum gastrin	390 pmol/L (normal <100 pmol/L)

Secretin test – intravenously 2 units GIH secretin per kg

Basal fasting value	401 pmol/L
10 min	265 pmol/L
20 min	280 pmol/L
30 min	300 pmol/L

a) What is the diagnosis?
1. Chronic pancreatitis
2. Gastrinoma
3. Retained gastric antrum
4. Ectopic gastrin secretion
5. Dumping syndrome

b) How would you confirm your diagnosis?
1. Ultrasound scan of abdomen
2. CT scan of abdomen
3. Angiography
4. At laparotomy
5. ERCP

Answer to Question 10 *is on page 192*

A 33-year-old male mechanic presents with a 6-month history of diarrhoea associated with crampy abdominal pain, lassitude, weight loss and a rash. He opens his bowels 8 times a day. He also has a pruritic rash over the elbows, which has persisted.

His father died in his 50s of lymphoma.

On examination he is apyrexial, has a pulse of 80/min, blood pressure of 120/60 mmHg, is cachectic +, and does not have lymphadenopathy. Abdominal examination reveals normal bowel sounds with some diffuse tenderness but no organomegaly; rectal examination is normal. He also has erythematous papules and plaques over the elbows, buttocks and knees.

INVESTIGATIONS

Hb	10.9 g/dL
MCV	94 fL
WCC	6.5×10^9/L
Platelets	247×10^9/L
Red cell folate	40 µgL
Vitamin B_{12}	200 pmol/L
TSH	3.8 mU/L
Free T4	12.9 nmol/L

a) What is the most likely diagnosis?
   1. Coeliac disease
   2. Giardiasis
   3. Crohn's disease
   4. Tropical sprue
   5. Common variable immunodeficiency

b) What is the most appropriate initial test?
   1. Hydrogen breath test
   2. Anti-tissue transglutaminase antibodies
   3. Immunoglobulin levels
   4. Small bowel follow-through
   5. Stool culture

c) What is the blood film not likely to show?
   1. Dimorphic picture
   2. Howell jolly bodies
   3. Acanthocytes
   4. Stomatocytes
   5. Target cells

Answer to Question 11 *is on page 193*

A 60-year-old male with type II diabetes controlled with diet and glicazide presents with a 4-day history of fever, myalgia and headache and a 2-day history of abdominal pain and diarrhoea. His wife called the GP when he became disorientated and confused. He had returned from a 2-week holiday in a new Spanish holiday complex 1 week before.

On examination his observations are: temperature 40°C: pulse 100/min regular, blood pressure 120/70 mmHg, respiration rate 24/min. He is disorientated and has mild neck stiffness but no other signs of meningism. Crackles are heard at his right base and in the left mid-zone on respiratory examination. Heart sounds are normal. There is diffuse abdominal tenderness and his liver edge can be felt two finger-breadths below the costal margin in the mid-clavicular line.

INVESTIGATIONS

Hb	13.5 g/dL
WBC	15 × 10^9/L - neutrophils 95%, lymphocytes 4%
Platelets	300 × 10^9/L
ESR	110 mm in the first hour
Sodium	127 mmol/L
Potassium	3.8 mmol/L
Urea	10.0 mmol/L
Creatinine	110 µmol/L
Albumin	38 g/L
Calcium	1.9 mmol/L
Phosphate	0.8 mmol/L
Bilirubin	14 µmol/L
Aspartate transaminase	80 iu/L
Alkaline phosphatase	200 iu/L
Glucose	5.0 mmol/L Hb A1c 7.5%
pH	7.4
PO$_2$	9.0 kPa
pCO$_2$	4.0 kPa
Chest X-ray	increased shadowing in the right base and a small pleural effusion
CSF	glucose 4.0 mmol/L, protein 0.45 g/L, <3 WBC/mm^3 no bacteria seen

Routine cultures of blood, urine, CSF, throat washings and stool are negative. The patient is started on intravenous amoxicillin but continues to deteriorate. He is switched to intravenous ceftriaxone.

Question continued overpage

a) What is the most likely diagnosis?
   1. Meningococcal sepsis
   2. *Legionella* pneumonia
   3. Pneumococcal pneumonia
   4. *Pseudomonas* infection
   5. *Pneumocystis carinii* pneumonia

b) His condition deteriorates further and he requires ventilation. Name two agents that should be added at this stage:
   1. Trimethoprim
   2. Erythromycin
   3. Rifampicin
   4. Augmentin
   5. Isoniazid
   6. Teicoplanin
   7. Flucloxacillin
   8. Amphotericin

Answer to Question 12 *is on page 195*

A 32-year-old air hostess presents with a 1-week history of fever and a migratory polyarthritis. For the last 2 days her left ankle and both knees have been painful and swollen but the other joints have settled. She has also developed pain in the dorsum of her left hand on movement. She takes the oral contraceptive pill only and has no known allergies.

On examination she has a hot swollen left ankle and left knee. She has several vesico-pustular lesions on her trunk, arms and lower legs.

INVESTIGATIONS

Hb	14.5 g/dL
WBC	12×10^9/L
Urea and electrolytes	normal
Rheumatoid factor	positive
Antinuclear factor	positive 1/100 homogenous
Synovial aspiration	turbid fluid containing 35 000 neutrophils/mL
Blood cultures	negative
Synovial fluid	negative

a) What is the most likely diagnosis?
   1. Rheumatoid arthritis
   2. Meningococcal arthritis
   3. Gout
   4. Gonococcal arthritis
   5. Acute psoriatic arthritis

b) Which of the following would you treat her with?
   1. Intravenous ceftriaxone
   2. Oral tetracycline
   3. Full dose non-steroidal antiinflammatory agent
   4. Oral prednisolone 30 mg
   5. Full dose colchicine

Answer to Question 13 *is on page 196*

Question 14

A 38-year-old Asian female presents with breathlessness, palpitations, a hoarse voice, sore throat and difficulty swallowing over the preceding week.

She is hypertensive and takes indapamide regularly. On examination her blood pressure is 130/70 mmHg and pulse 130/min irregular. She is apyrexial and comfortable at rest.

Blood results show:

Hb	13.4 g/dL
WCC	18 × 10⁹/L
Sodium	130 mmol/L
Potassium	3.2 mmol/L
Urea	7.8 mmol/L
Creatinine	85 µmol/L
ESR	80 mm/h
TSH	0.05 mU/L, fT4 53.4 pmol/L

a) What is the most likely cause of the abnormal results?
1. De Quervains thyroiditis
2. Sick Euthyroidism
3. Grave's disease
4. Toxic adenoma
5. TSH secreting pituitary adenoma

b) What would a Technetium thyroid isotope uptake scan show?
1. Diffuse uptake
2. Reduced uptake
3. Patchy irregular uptake
4. A cold nodule
5. A warm nodule

Answer to Question 14 *is on page 197*

A 17-year-old female is reviewed 6-monthly, having been treated for acute lymphocytic leukaemia 10 years previously. She has recently returned from Greece where she has been living for the past 2 years. She presents with a 6-month history of 8 kg weight loss, general malaise, and amenorrhoea. On examination she is obviously thin, has downy hair over her face and neck, and has cool peripheries. There is no lymphadenopathy. Cardiovascular, respiratory and abdominal examinations are otherwise normal.

Full blood count, urea, electrolytes and liver function tests are all normal.

What is the most likely diagnosis?

1. Recurrent leukaemia
2. Anorexia nervosa
3. Tuberculosis
4. Secondary malignancy
5. Brucellosis

A 50-year-old female was seen in the emergency department with a recurrence of acute sinus pain. On direct questioning she had had a number of episodes of diarrhoea in the past 2–3 years. These had successfully been treated by her GP with metronidazole. Her childhood had been characterized by numerous chest infections. She was not on regular medication and had never smoked or drunk alcohol.

Examination reveals evidence of a right otitis media. On auscultation of the chest there are coarse crackles in the right lower lobe. On palpation of her abdomen a splenic tip is palpable. The cardiovascular system and central nervous system are normal.

INVESTIGATIONS

Hb	12 g/dL
WBC	4.0×10^9/L – 55% neutrophils, 40% lymphocytes
Platelets	200×10^9/L
ESR	15 mm in the first hour
Sodium	135 mmol/L
Potassium	4.0 mmol/L
Urea	5.0 mmol/L
Creatinine	105 µmol/L
Albumin	43 g/L
Total protein	60 g/L
Aspartate aminotransferase	20 iu/L
Alkaline phosphatase	90 iu/L
Bilirubin	6 µmol/L
Rheumatoid factor and ANA	negative
Cultures of blood and stool	negative
Chest X-ray	normal
Abdominal ultrasound	splenomegaly

a) What is the most likely diagnosis?
1. Cystic fibrosis
2. Complement deficiency
3. Common variable immunodeficiency
4. Chronic granulomatous disease
5. Chiadek Higashi syndrome

b) What investigation would you request?
1. Sweat test
2. Complement function
3. Barium follow through
4. Neutrophil function
5. Immunoglobulin levels

Answer to Question 16 *is on page 200*

A 38-year-old female visits her GP for a routine health check. She has been fit and well.

The lab posts the following results:

Hb	11.2 g/dL
WCC	6.8×10^9/L
Platelets	183×10^9/L
MCV	65.2 fL
MCH	19.6 pg
Reticulocytes	50×10^9/L
ESR	10 mm in first hour
Serum ferritin	56 ug/L

Which diagnosis is most likely?

1. Haemoglobin H disease
2. Beta-thalassaemia minor
3. Latent iron deficiency
4. Congenital sideroblastic anaemia
5. Idiopathic haemochromatosis

A 58-year-old farmer complains of breathlessness and a dry cough that has worsened gradually over 3 months. Recently he has found working difficult because of dyspnoea and is considering retiring. He has occasional mild fevers and influenza-like symptoms and had lost 3 kg in weight. Generally all of his symptoms are worse towards the end of the day. He had an anterior myocardial infarct 5 years previously, complicated by left ventricular failure, but this is now well controlled with an angiotensin converting enzyme inhibitor, a beta blocker and diuretics. He gave up smoking after his myocardial infarction.

On examination he is not cyanosed or clubbed. Jugular venous pressure is normal and his blood pressure is 150/70 mmHg. On auscultation there are fine inspiratory crackles heard in both lung bases.

INVESTIGATIONS

Hb	13.9 g/dL
WBC	10×10^9/L
ESR	50 mm in the first hour
Sodium	137 mmol/L
Potassium	3.9 mmol/L
Urea	8 mmol/L
Albumin	43 g/L
Total protein	78 g/L
Aspartate transaminase	35 iu/L
Alkaline phosphatase	111 iu/L
Bilirubin	12 μmol/L
RF	positive
ANA	negative

The ECG is unremarkable aside from changes consistent with old myocardial infarction. A chest X-ray shows areas of nodular shadowing in both lung bases.

FEV1 70%, FVC 80%, DLCO 70%, KCO 60%. Arterial oxygen saturation is 96% at rest and 92% on walking 100 m.

a) Given the history and above findings what is the most likely diagnosis?
1. Idiopathic pulmonary fibrosis
2. Lymphangitis carcinomatosis
3. *Pneumocystis carinii* pneumonia
4. Extrinsic allergic alveolitis
5. Histiocytosis-X

Question continued overpage

b) Broncho-alveolar lavage analysis would show:
1. An elevated lymphocyte count with CD4>CD8
2. A low lymphocyte count
3. An elevated lymphocyte count with CD8>CD4
4. Malignant cells
5. *Pneumocystis carinii*

Answer to Question 18 *is on page 203*

A 57-year-old engineer has recently retired early because of fatigue and shortness of breath. He has been a lifelong non-smoker. A chest X-ray performed 2 months earlier showed no abnormality and he was commenced on a low dose of furosemide, which has had no effect. A repeat chest X-ray demonstrates a large right-sided pleural effusion.

These are the blood results received from the GP:

Hb	12.2 g/dL
WCC	12.1 × 10⁹/L
Platelets	154 × 10⁹/L
Sodium	130 mmol/L
Potassium	3.2 mmol/L
Urea	7.8 mmol/L
Creatinine	134 μmol/L
CaCorr	3.0 mmol/L
Albumin	23 g/L
Alkaline phosphatase	45 iu/L
Phosphate	1.38 mmol/L
Bicarbonate	35 mmol/L

What is the most likely cause of the above results?

1. Mesothelioma
2. Hyperparathyroidoism
3. Squamous cell carcinoma
4. Metastatic oat cell carcinoma
5. Asbestosis

A 50-year-old Asian male presents with a week of cough, chest pain, fever, night sweats and anorexia. A chest film reveals consolidation at the apices and a cavity in the left upper lobe. Sputum microscopy reveals the presence of acid-fast bacilli. A Heaf test has shown a grade 2 response.

The patient takes azathioprine and prednisolone for a renal allograft performed 7 months ago. His creatinine is 110 umol/L.

The treatment of choice should be:

1. Isoniazid, rifampacin and pyrazinamide
2. Isoniazid, rifampacin, pyrazinamide and ethambutol
3. Rifampacin, pyrazinamide and ethambutol
4. Isoniazid, rifampacin, pyrazinamide, ethambutol and streptomycin
5. Await culture and sensitivity before starting an appropriate regimen

A 50-year-old female has had a long history of abdominal cramps and diarrhoea. She has lost weight. Her previous history includes pelvic radio-therapy for carcinoma of the ovary.

Her blood results are as follows:

Hb	10.2 g/dL
WCC	8.9×10^9/L
Platelets	202×10^9/L
MCV	110 fL
Vitamin B_{12}	96 ng/L
Serum Folate	20 µg/L
Calcium	2.4 mmol/L
Phosphate	1.0 mmol/L
Urea and electrolytes	normal
Liver function tests	normal

Which of the following would be the most useful initial test?

1. Small bowel biopsy
2. Abdominal ultrasound
3. Small bowel barium meal
4. Schilling test
5. 14C xylose breath test

Answer to Question 21 *is on page 207*

A 17-year-old female presents with jaundice, having taken an overdose of 30 paracetamol tablets 36 h previously.

a) What is the best test to ascertain her prognosis and treatment?
  1. Paracetamol level
  2. AST
  3. Serial measurements of mental state
  4. Urinary bilirubin levels
  5. Caffeine clearance
  6. Prothrombin time

Twenty four hours later you are contacted by the junior team member because she has become mildly confused and you are told that her blood gases show a pH of 7.42, her INR is 1.6, her creatinine has risen to 122 μmol/L, and she has serum glucose of 3.8 mmol/L.

b) What would be your management?
  1. Refer urgently for liver transplantation
  2. Continue N-acetylcysteine infusions and monitor closely
  3. Arrange for haemodialysis
  4. Commence bicarbonate infusion
  5. Commence an infusion of 50 mL 50% dextrose

A 65-year-old male presents complaining of bilateral leg weakness. Over the previous 3 months he has felt tired, lost 5 kg in weight and has developed upper and mid-back pain which now radiates round to his nipples and has required regular codeine phosphate. Recently he developed night sweats that resolved after he was given a short course of antibiotics for a presumed urinary tract infection. His wife (a retired district nurse) has also been giving him glycerol suppositories for constipation.

On examination he is cachectic, alert and orientated. His temperature is 37.5°C. He has tender thoracic and lumbar vertebrae. Hip and knee flexion is weak bilaterally. Light touch and pinprick are reduced in both lower limbs with a sensory level at the nipples. Vibration sense and proprioception were reduced in both feet. The tendon reflexes are present and equal. The plantar reflexes are extensor on both sides. Per rectum examination is normal (normal tone, contraction and prostate).

INVESTIGATIONS

Hb	14 g/L
WBC	8×10^9/L
Platelets	450×10^9/L
ESR	17 mm in the first hour
Sodium	140 mmol/L
Potassium	4 mmol/L
Urea	6.5 mmol/L
CRP	10 mg/L
Aspartate aminotransferase	27 iu/L
Alkaline phosphatase	170 iu/L
Creatine phosphokinase	20 iu/L
PSA	normal
Chest X-ray lung fields	clear

The 4th and 5th thoracic vertebrae are sclerotic and reduced in height; there is loss of the intervertebral disc space.

ECG sinus rhythm 76, normal axis.

a) What is the most likely diagnosis?
  1. Multiple sclerosis
  2. Guillane–Barré syndrome
  3. Bony metastases with spinal cord compression
  4. Spinal osteomyelitis with spinal cord compression
  5. Polymyositis

Question continued overpage

b) The three most important investigations are:
1. Blood cultures
2. CSF examination
3. MRI scan of thoracic spine
4. MRI scan of brain
5. Echocardiogram
6. CT guided biopsy of affected vertebrae
7. Nerve conduction studies
8. MRI scan of lumbar spine

Answer to Question 23 *is on page 210*

A female who is 19 weeks pregnant presents to the emergency department in an anxious state because she has just been to a party where a child was noted to have chickenpox. She and her mother are unsure whether she has previously been affected by chickenpox.

What action would you take?

1. Send her blood sample to the nearest virology lab. If she has antibodies she is immune and no further action need be taken
2. Give her 1 g of zoster immune globulin immediately
3. Reassure her that there is no appreciable risk to the fetus
4. Commence a prophylactic course of oral acyclovir
5. Review in 1 week to see whether she has contracted chicken pox and treat if necessary

A 20-year-old female is known to have sickle cell disease. She is admitted with a 2-day history of cough, intermittent fever and pleuritic chest pain. One week previously she had been to the emergency department with low back pain and had been given opiate analgesia and a prescription for naproxen. In the past she has had similar episodes and 6 months before admission she was treated for pain in the hips and legs after cycling in cold weather.

On examination she is hypoxic (O_2 saturation 87%) and in obvious distress. Her temperature is 38.2°C. On examination of the respiratory system there are some scattered crepitations at the left base. The chest X-ray shows bilateral patchy infiltration in both lung fields.

Which would you consider to be **least** appropriate in this patient's current and future management?

1. Broad spectrum antibiotics
2. Exchange transfusion
3. Allopurinol
4. Hydroxyurea
5. Pneumococcal vaccination

Answer to Question 25 *is on page 212*

A 30-year-old male smoker presents with a long history of abdominal pain and diarrhoea. Over the last week he has developed some painful red marks over his legs. He also complains of persistent back pain and stiffness, which is worse in the morning.

Examination confirms red, hot and tender lesions distributed over his shins. Rectal examination reveals a single ulcer and purple skin tag. The remainder of the examination is unremarkable.

Which of the following statements is correct?

1. Ulcerative colitis is more likely then Crohn's disease
2. Barium follow through may show fistulas and skip lesions
3. The rash is more likely to be pyoderma gangrenosum
4. He is likely to be HLA DR3 positive
5. Infliximab may be commenced to control his symptoms

A 35-year-old male is referred with gynaecomastia and infertility. He recently tripped over and fractured his forearm.

INVESTIGATIONS

Testosterone	5.8 nmol/L	9–24
LH	20.1 u/L	3–10
FSH	28 u/L	3–10

a) What is the likely diagnosis?
   1. Klinefelter's syndrome
   2. Kallman's syndrome
   3. Noonan's syndrome
   4. Marfan's syndrome
   5. Turner's syndrome

b) What would be the most appropriate test to confirm the diagnosis?
   1. Short synacthen test
   2. Testicular biopsy
   3. MRI pituitary
   4. Buccal smear
   5. Lymphocyte karyotyping

Answer to Question 27 *is on page 216*

Which one of the following statements is true regarding hypercalcaemia?

1. Hyperparathyroidism is the commonest cause in hospitalized patients
2. It is often difficult to distinguish the humoral hypercalcemia of malignancy from primary hyperparathyroidism, because typically the serum calcium level and the parathyroid hormone level will be high in both disorders
3. Hypercalcaemia due to malignancy is often associated with a hyperchloraemic metabolic acidosis
4. May be treated with intravenous saline and thiazide diuretics
5. Pamidronate is effective in cases of hypercalcaemia associated with malignancy

Answer to Question 28 *is on page 218*

A 20-year-old male is admitted with severe abdominal pain, vomiting and constipation. He has a history of previous admissions with similar symptoms. During this episode he has noticed a raised non-pruritic lesion on the back of his hand. Similar lesions had been noted at various sites in the past.

On examination his abdomen is distended but not tender. A plain abdominal X-ray shows several fluid levels in the small bowel.

a) What is the most likely diagnosis?
1. Amyloidosis
2. Sarcoidosis
3. Acute intermittent porphyria
4. Chronic urticaria
5. C1-esterase inhibitor deficiency

b) Which one investigation would you first request?
1. Urinary aminovulinic acid and porphobilinogen
2. Measure C3 level
3. Skin prick testing
4. Allergy testing
5. Rectal biopsy
6. Measure C4 level
7. Mast cell tryptase

c) Which one treatment may be of benefit for this patient to prevent further attacks?
1. Antihistamines
2. Danazol
3. Bromocryptine
4. Non-steroidal antiinflammatory agents
5. Intramuscular adrenaline (epinephrine) (epipen)
6. Oral steroids
7. Colchicine

Answer to Question 29 *is on page 219*

A 55-year-old unemployed male waiter is referred from the GP with increasing shortness of breath over 3–4 months associated with a dry non-productive cough. He has been a lifelong non-smoker and keeps no pets. He takes no medication other than an occasional paracetamol. His past history is unremarkable aside from childhood asthma which now rarely bothers him.

On examination his temperature is 36.2°C, pulse 78/min and blood pressure 120/70 mmHg. He has marked clubbing and a degree of cyanosis. There are no palpable lymph nodes. Examination of the chest reveals bilateral mid to late inspiratory crepitations heard from the bases to the mid-zones. The remainder of the examination is normal.

Blood results are as follows:

Hb	12.6 g/dL
WBC	10.2 10^9/L
Neutrophils	7.2 × 10^9/L
Lymphocytes	1.4 × 10^9/L
Eosinophils	0.6 × 10^9/L
Urea	8.4 mmol/L
Creatinine	104 µmol/L
Urinalysis	Normal
Chest X-ray	Reticular nodular shadowing in the lower zones

Lung function test results:

FEV1	1.84 L
FVC	2.04 L
FEV1/FVC	90%
TLC	2.95 L
RV	1.7 L
TLCO	38 % predicted
KCO	58 % predicted

a) What do the lung function tests show?
   1. A restrictive pattern
   2. Indicative of airways obstruction
   3. Restrictive lung defect with reduced gas transfer
   4. Mixed restrictive and obstructive picture
   5. Pleural thickening

b) What would be the next appropriate test to reach a diagnosis?
   1. High resolution CT thorax
   2. Transbronchial lung biopsy
   3. Gallium scanning
   4. Serum ACE level
   5. Autoantibody screen

Question continued overpage

c) What is the likely diagnosis in this case?
   1. Extrinsic allergic alveolitis
   2. Idiopathic pulmonary fibrosis
   3. Acute sarcoidosis
   4. Mesothelioma
   5. Churg Strauss syndrome

Answer to Question 30 *is on page 220*

A 45-year-old male presented to the rheumatology clinic with painful knees. Past medical history included meningococcal meningitis at the age of 20 and gonorrhoea at the age of 24. He had otherwise enjoyed good health until 2 years before admission when he became impotent, which had led to marital difficulties. He smoked 20 cigarettes a day and drank 4 pints of beer per night when on leave in the UK.

On examination he looks well with a marked suntan, having recently returned from Saudi Arabia where he worked as an engineer. Marked crepitus is present in both knees. He has a large tense right knee effusion and a moderate left knee effusion. His testes are small and his pubic hair is sparse.

INVESTIGATIONS

Hb	14 g/dL
WBC	5 × 10⁹/L
ESR	15 mm in the first hour
Urea and electrolytes	normal
Urine dipstick	glucose ++

a) What is the cause of the arthritis?
   1. Osteoarthritis
   2. Gout
   3. Chondrocalcinosis
   4. Osteomyelitis
   5. Reactive arthritis

b) What is the likely diagnosis?
   1. Alcoholic liver disease
   2. Prolactinoma
   3. Haemochromatosis
   4. Wilson's disease
   5. Whipple's disease

Answer to Question 31 *is on page 221*

An alcoholic with known oesophageal and gastric varices is admitted with haematemesis. He undergoes emergency endoscopy that shows an oesophageal variceal bleed for which he has variceal band ligation. The second day after admission he has a further bleed and after transfusion he is currently haemodynamically stable.

Which of the following would now be most appropriate?

1. Balloon tamponade
2. Transjugular intrahepatic stent shunt insertion
3. Glypressin infusion
4. Variceal sclerotherapy
5. Repeat variceal band ligation

A 25-year-old male complained of muscle cramps, which prevented him from playing football. He had always experienced muscle pain during the initial period of exercise but found that his symptoms passed off with continued graduated exertion. He was otherwise fit and well and there was no relevant family history. General examination was unremarkable and neurologically he had no evidence of muscle weakness.

Baseline investigations including muscle enzymes and an EMG were normal. An ischaemic forearm test was performed which demonstrated no rise in the venous lactate level after cessation of exercise.

a) What is the likely diagnosis?
1. Hypokalaemic periodic paralysis
2. Von Gierke's disease
3. McArdle's disease
4. Pompe's disease
5. Gaucher's disease

b) How would you confirm this?
1. β-glucocerebrosidase levels
2. Alpha glucosidase levels
3. Glucose 6 phosphatase levels
4. Muscle phosphorylase levels
5. Serum potassium levels

Answer to Question 33 *is on page 224*

A 31-year-old female is awaiting surgery for a phaeochromocytoma. You are called to the ward to find her sweating profusely.

   Observations: pulse 50/min and blood pressure 220/170 mmHg.

What therapy would you institute?

1. IV atropine
2. IV phentolamine
3. IV fluids and close observation
4. IV hydralazine
5. IV propanolol

Answer to Question 34 *is on page 225*

A 30-year-old obese female presents to the diabetic clinic. She has had problems with her glucose control despite close attention to her diet and regular review in the clinic. She is currently taking metformin: 850 mg 12 hourly. She had previously tried a combination of metformin and gliclazide but this has led to weight gain.

INVESTIGATIONS

Urine dip	negative
Blood pressure	120/70
Previous renal function tests	normal
HbA_{IC}	7.8%

What treatment would you consider?

1. Recommend commencing an insulin regimen
2. Change to rosiglitazone
3. Increase dose of metformin
4. Add rosiglitazone in combination with metformin
5. None of the above

A 10-year-old Asian female attended hospital complaining of a 10-day history of fever and malaise. Her ankles, right wrist and left knee had been stiff and painful for 5 days. Her GP had seen her 2 weeks previously and given her a course of antibiotics for a sore throat and mild upper respiratory tract infection. She was treated with aspirin, following which her fever settled over 48 h and her joints became much less painful.

She had no previous history of joint problems. Twelve weeks before, she had returned from a 6-week holiday in Pakistan, where both she and her brother had contracted hepatitis. She had been immunized against tuberculosis at the age of 9.

On examination, her temperature is 39°C and there is no pharyngitis, no lymphadenopathy and no rashes. Her pulse is 90/min regular, jugular venous pressure is not elevated, and there are normal first and second heart sounds and a soft pericardial rub. She does not have hepatosplenomegaly. The joints are painful and swollen.

INVESTIGATIONS

Hb	10 g/L
MCV	80 fL
WBC	12×10^9/L 70% neutrophils
Platelets	400×10^9/L
Haemoglobin electrophoresis	normal
Urea and electrolytes	normal
Bilirubin	7 mmol/L
Aspartate aminotransferase	65 iu/L
ESR	115 mm in the first hour
Latex and autoantibody screen	negative
IgG	25 g/L
IgA	3.14 g/L
IgM	2.11 g/L
C-reactive protein	80 mg/L
Cultures of blood, urine and throat	negative
Paul–Bunnell	negative
Hepatitis B Ag	negative
Hepatitis A antibodies – acute serum	1/1280, convalescent serum 1/640
ASO titre	500 iu/L

Left knee aspirate of 20 mL of yellow fluid containing 3000 neutrophils/mL is sterile on culture. Urinalysis shows a trace of protein but no casts or cells on microscopy. Nothing abnormal was detected on a chest X-ray and X-rays of the affected joints. ECG sinus rhythm, PR interval 0.3 ms, normal axis, normal QRS echocardiogram – mild mitral regurgitation, small pericardial effusion.

Question continued overpage

What is the most likely cause of her clinical picture?

1. Group A beta haemolytic streptococcal infection
2. Hepatitis A infection
3. Systemic lupus erythematosus
4. Infective endocarditis
5. Still's disease

Answer to Question 36 *is on page 228*

A 35-year-old bisexual HIV positive male is on treatment with highly active anti-retroviral therapy (HAART). His recent CD4 count was 500 cells/μL and he has an undetectable viral load.

He has a new female partner who is unaware of the diagnosis and he wishes to start a family.

Which of the following is true?

1. If they conceive and she is HIV positive the risk of vertical transmission is 80%
2. She is entitled to know his HIV status
3. You must tell her his HIV status immediately to prevent infection
4. Sexual intercourse is safe if limited to the fertile period
5. You may not breach his confidentiality at any stage

Answer to Question 37 *is on page 229*

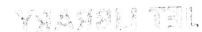

A 53-year-old female with breast cancer has an indwelling line for treatment and has just had a course of chemotherapy. Following the treatment her platelets remain low despite multiple HLA matched transfusions and a return of her normal red and white cell counts. Her medication was withheld but the thrombocytopenia has persisted.

Examination reveals palatal and lower limb petechiae but no organomegaly.

Blood results are as follows:

Hb	11.2 g/dL	
WCC	7.6 (67% neutrophils, 20% lymphocytes)	
MCV	81 fL	
Platelets	5 ×10⁹/L	
Mean platelet volume	11.2 fL	6.2–10.6
Coagulation	normal	
Urea and electrolytes	normal	
Blood film	no platelet clumping, no shistocytes	

What is the most likely diagnosis?

1. Disseminated intravascular coagulation
2. Iatrogenic myelosuppression
3. Aplastic anaemia
4. Hypersplenism secondary to metastatic infiltration
5. Immune-mediated thrombocytopenia

JET LIBRARY

A 29-year-old non-smoking Japanese female presents to casualty with sudden onset right pleuritic chest pain and shortness of breath. She has a large right pneumothorax that is treated appropriately. On review in the outpatient department she reports a gradual but progressive deterioration in her exercise tolerance that preceded the pneumothorax. She denies any other symptoms. Chest X-ray shows full re-expansion of the right lung but the radiologist reports reticulonodular changes at both bases that, in hindsight, were present on her initial chest X-ray. A CT scan shows diffuse cystic change at the lung bases and a small left pleural effusion. Clinical examination is normal.

The most likely diagnosis is:

1. Neurofibromatosis
2. Langerhan's cell histiocytosis
3. Lymphangiomyomatosis
4. Hermansky Pudlak syndrome
5. Alveolar proteinosis

Answer to Question 39 *is on page 232*

A 26-year-old female attends her GP with cystitis, for which he prescribes an empirical course of trimethoprim. Five days later her symptoms persist and she complains of nausea and occasional vomiting. In addition to sending an MSU for culture, the GP checks her serum biochemistry, the results of which are:

Sodium	138 mmol/L
Potassium	4.4 mmol/L
Bicarbonate	21 mmol/L
Urea	5.6 mmol/L
Creatinine	183 μmol/L

What is the likely explanation for the patient's biochemical abnormality?

1. Pregnancy
2. Vomiting
3. Iatrogenic
4. Racial origin
5. Rhabdomyolysis

Answer to Question 40 *is on page 234*

The following is a series of excerpts from a 24-h tape (lead V1).

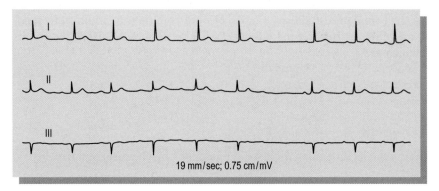

19 mm/sec; 0.75 cm/mV

What is demonstrated?

1. Complete heart block
2. Wenkebach phenomenon
3. Mobitz type II
4. Junctional escape rhythm
5. Trifascicular block

A 46-year-old male with a history of alcohol abuse is admitted with progressive left thigh swelling and abnormal purpuric lesions over that area. There was no history of trauma.

On examination he is jaundiced and has 4-cm hepatomegaly. His left thigh is obviously swollen and tender with confluent non-blanching rash. There is no evidence of an underlying haematoma.

Blood results are as follows:

Hb	9.5 g/dL
Platelets	120 × 10⁹/L
MCV	100 fL
WCC	8.7 × 10⁹/L
INR	1.2
APPT	36.1 s Control 34 s

Which of the following would be most likely to account for his presentation?

1. Vitamin E deficiency
2. Vitamin A deficiency
3. Vitamin C deficiency
4. Vitamin K deficiency
5. Niacin deficiency

A middle-aged female is referred with thirst, polydipsia and polyuria. She was involved in a road traffic accident 9 months before admission and thought her symptoms had begun soon after this. She had had no serious illness in the past and took no medication.

General examination is normal, her blood pressure is 120/80 mmHg and there is no postural drop. Her 24-h urine collections are between 7 and 12 L.

INVESTIGATIONS

Sodium	130 mmol/L
Potassium	3.5 mmol/L
Urea	2.0 mmol/L
Glucose	5 mmol/L
Protein	70 g/L
Albumin	35 g/L
Alkaline phosphatase	80 iu/L
Bilirubin	5 μmol/L
Plasma osmolality	268 mOsmol/kg
Urine osmolality	50 mOsmol/kg

a) What is the likely diagnosis?
   1. Inappropriate anti-diuretic hormone secretion
   2. Psychogenic polydipsia
   3. Diuretic abuse
   4. Neurogenic diabetes insipidus
   5. Nephrogenic diabetes insipidus

b) What investigation would you arrange?
   1. Measurement of anti-diuretic hormone levels
   2. Repeat plasma and urine osmolality
   3. Water deprivation test
   4. CT scan of head
   5. Urinary sodium

Answer to Question 43 *is on page 238*

A 14-year-old Caucasian male presented to the emergency department with headache, photophobia, neck stiffness and a purpuric rash. His condition has deteriorated and for the last 4 days he has been intubated in the intensive care department. He had been admitted previously with a similar problem. His parents indicate that one of his other relatives had survived a similar illness.

What one investigation would you do to reach an underlying diagnosis?

1. CH50 total haemolytic complement assay
2. C3 and C4
3. Immunoglobulins
4. Nitroblue tetrazolium test
5. CD3, -4, -8, -19 lymphocyte markers

Answer to Question 44 *is on page 240*

A 33-year-old housewife presents with fatigue, weakness and weight gain. 5 months previously her menstrual periods had stopped. Her GP found her to be hypertensive and commenced a thiazide diuretic. Two weeks after starting she developed polyuria. Her GP dipped her urine, which showed +++ for glucose. He then referred her to the clinic where the clinic sister recorded a BM reading of 8.4.

On examination she: is mildly obese, has facial hair, has thin extremities, her pulse is 80/min, her blood pressure is 174/94 mmHg and her temperature is 36.2°C. There is no thyroid enlargement and she has generalized proximal weakness – she is unable to stand from a squatting position. Three 24-h urine cortisol levels are all elevated.

Which investigation would you next organize to try and achieve a diagnosis?

1. Fasting glucose
2. Basal cortisol level
3. Plasma ACTH levels
4. Low and high dexamethosone suppression tests
5. Abdominal CT

A 60-year-old female presented with abdominal pain. She had been unwell for 2–3 weeks and felt 'weak'. For 3 weeks she had had intermittent sharp pains in her left upper quadrant and more recently a dull ache in her left iliac fossa. A week before admission she developed night sweats. There had been several episodes when she had become dizzy and confused and on one occasion she had lost vision in her left eye. She had a number of vague rheumatic symptoms but no early morning stiffness, headaches or jaw claudication. In the past she had had a hysterectomy and a cholecystectomy. She took no regular medication. There was no family history of significant disease.

On examination observations are: temperature 39°C, pulse 120/min, blood pressure 140/60 mmHg, respiratory rate 40/min. She has no rash, lymphadenopathy or clubbing. Two small conjunctival haemorrhages are visible. Examination of her respiratory system is unremarkable. Her heart sounds are normal; a soft pansystolic murmur can be heard only at the apex. There is a tender pulsatile mass in the left iliac fossa and the spleen is palpable and tender. Neurological examination is normal. The peripheral pulses are present and equal. There are no bruits.

INVESTIGATIONS

Hb	11 g/dL
WBC	8.0×10^9/L
Platelets	300×10^9/L
ESR	50 mm in the first hour
Sodium	140 mmol/L
Potassium	4.0 mmol/L
Urea	9 mmol/L
Creatinine	90 µmol/L
Albumin	30 g/L
Bilirubin	8.0 µmol/L
Aspartate aminotransferase	40 iu/L
Alkaline phosphatase	140 iu/l
Calcium	2.0 mmol/L
Chest X-ray and abdominal X-rays	normal
ECG	sinus tachycardia
Urinalysis	protein +, blood +, no casts seen
Serial blood cultures	no growth reported

An ultrasound of the abdomen shows a large spleen with wedge-shaped areas of increased density.

Question continued overpage

a) What is the most likely diagnosis?
1. Diverticular abcess
2. Metastatic carcinoma of colon
3. Infective endocarditis
4. Rheumatoid arthritis
5. Lymphoma

b) Suggest the most appropriate next investigation:
1. CT chest abdomen and pelvis
2. Bone marrow aspirate and trephine
3. CT enema
4. Echocardiogram
5. Digital subtraction angiography of iliac vessels

Answer to Question 46 *is on page 243*

A 68-year-old builder is referred with a history of easy fatigue, macroscopic haematuria and symptoms suggestive of acrocyanosis.

Examination was unremarkable aside from a palpable splenic tip.

INVESTIGATIONS

Hb	10.5 g/dL
Reticulocyte count	2.4% (0.5–2.5%)
Urine microscopy	no intact red cells
Blood film	marked autoagglutination; spherocytes present

a) What is the most likely diagnosis?
  1. Cryoglobulinaemia
  2. Warm autoimmune haemolytic anaemia
  3. Hereditary spherocytosis
  4. Paroxysmal nocturnal haemoglobinaemia
  5. Cold autoimmune haemolytic anaemia

b) In this patient which of the following is most likely to be true?
  1. The direct antiglobulin (Coombs) test is likely to be positive for complement only
  2. Treatment with Methyldopa could produce this clinical state
  3. A myeloma screen should routinely be performed
  4. The direct antiglobulin test is likely to be negative
  5. The diagnosis may be confirmed with the Hams acid lysis test

Answer to Question 47 *is on page 245*

A 50-year-old female with chronic asthma is admitted with nausea and vomiting and shortness of breath. She had been treated with erythromycin by her GP for a chest infection as she was allergic to penicillin. Her usual medication is a long acting beta-2 agonist, an inhaled steroid and theophylline.

On examination she is shaking and anxious but able to complete full sentences. She has a respiration rate of 28/min, pulse of 120/min, blood pressure 140/70 mmHg and temperature of 36°C. O_2 saturation 97% on air. Examination of her chest reveals equal air entry with little evidence of wheeze. Her peak flow is 400 (best 450).

Blood gases (on air) were taken in casualty:

pH	7.36
PO_2	11.4 kPa
PCO_2	4.3 kPa
HCO_3	25 mmol/L

a) What is the likely cause of her symptoms?
1. Hyperventilation
2. Overuse of beta-2 agonist
3. Pulmonary embolus
4. Acute severe asthma
5. Theophylline toxicity

b) The most important test performed in casualty would now be:
1. CRP
2. Serum potassium
3. Repeat blood gases
4. Chest X-ray
5. Paracetamol level

Answer to Question 48 *is on page 247*

A 52-year-old male has a non-productive cough and exertional breathlessness. He has also had feverish symptoms and malaise, and has lost 7 kg over the previous 6 weeks. He has a history of mild asthma but is not on current medication. He is a non-smoker.

The most marked abnormality on a chest X-ray is the presence of peripheral lung infiltrates.

INVESTIGATIONS

Hb	14 g/dL
WCC	10×10^9 /L(40% polymorphs, 15% lymphocytes)
Platelets	160×10^9/L
Urea and electrolytes	normal
Liver function tests	normal
CRP	15 mg/L
ESR	30 mm/hr

The most likely diagnosis is:

1. Idiopathic pulmonary fibrosis
2. Histiocytosis X
3. Chronic eosinophilic pneumonia
4. Lymphangiomyomatosis
5. Loeffler's syndrome (simple pulmonary eosinophilia)

Answer to Question 49 *is on page 248*

A 32-year-old female presents with a 2-month history of jaundice after starting the oral contraceptive pill and 1 month after returning from Turkey, where she had contracted a short-lived illness, characterized by fever and diarrhoea. She had felt run down for several months and attributed this to working long hours as a barmaid.

While sunbathing in Turkey, she had noticed several painless patches on her hands and face, which did not tan. She takes no regular medication. She is a non-smoker and drinks between 2 and 3 glasses of wine per day. On examination she has depigmented areas on both hands and on her face. She is icteric and several spider naevi are noted. The remainder of her examination is normal.

INVESTIGATIONS

Hb	12 g/L
WBC	8 × 10⁹/L
Platelets	150 × 10⁹/L
MCV	99 fL
Bilirubin	90 μmol/L
Alamine aminotransferase	185 iu/L
Alkaline phosphatase	200 iu/L
Total protein	80 g/L
Albumin	26 g/L
HBS Ag	negative
Hep A serology	positive 1/640
Rheumatoid factor	negative
ANA positive	1/160

*Handwritten annotations: "↑↑ er Globulinaemia *" next to Albumin; ANA positive marked with asterisk*

a) What is the most likely diagnosis?
   1. Autoimmune chronic active hepatitis
   2. Drug-induced hepatitis (oral contraceptive pill)
   3. Primary biliary cirrhosis
   4. Primary sclerosing cholangitis
   5. Systemic lupus erythematosus

b) Which of the following investigations is likely to be positive?
   1. Anti mitochondrial antibodies
   2. Alpha-1-antitrypsin
   3. Anti-smooth muscle antibodies and anti-liver-kidney microsomes (LKMI)
   4. Serum caeruloplasmin and urinary copper
   5. Cholangiography

Question continued overpage

c) Which of the following is the first line treatment?
1. Interferon therapy
2. Corticosteroids
3. Lamivudine
4. Azathioprine
5. Cyclophosphamide

A 78-year-old patient presents with breathlessness that had been exacerbated by gardening. You are shown her ECG while she is being triaged in the emergency department

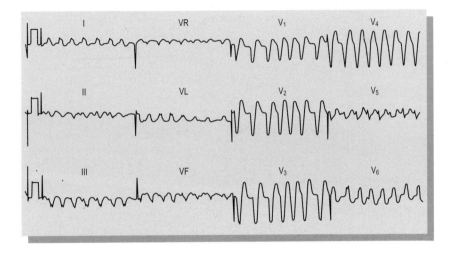

What does the ECG show?

1. Atrial fibrillation with right bundle branch block
2. Left bundle branch block
3. Atrial flutter with 2:1 block
4. Ventricular tachycardia
5. Atrial fibrillation with left bundle branch block

Answer to Question 5 I *is on page 252*

Question 52

A 26-year-old female presents to casualty after a series of grand mal fits. She had been well until the onset of fits 12 h previously. On examination she has a temperature of 38°C, pulse 90/min and blood pressure 135/90 mmHg. Neurologically she is alert but has a left VI cranial nerve palsy and upper motor neurone weakness of the right arm.

INVESTIGATIONS

Hb	9.7 g/dL
WBC	8.9 × 10⁹/L
Platelets	20 × 10⁹/L
Blood film	red cell fragmentation
PT	12 s
APTT	34 s
Fibrinogen	2.5 g/L
TT	18 s
Sodium	134 mmol/L
Potassium	5.2 mmol/L
Urea	26 mmol/L
Creatinine	364 µmol/L
Urine microscopy	blood ++, protein ++

What is the likely diagnosis?

1. Sepsis with disseminated intravascular coagulation
2. Systemic lupus erythematosus with idiopathic thrombocytopenia purpura
3. Thrombotic thrombocytopenic purpura
4. Haemolytic uraemic syndrome
5. Malignant hypertension

Answer to Question 52 *is on page 253*

A 45-year-old smoker complains of tiredness and weakness.

INVESTIGATIONS

Blood pressure	180/110 mmHg
Sodium	140 mmol/L
Potassium	2.8 mmol/L
Bicarbonate	32 mmol/L
Urea	5 mmol/L
Glucose	12 mmol/L

What is the likely diagnosis?

1. Type II diabetes
2. Addison's disease
3. Oat cell carcinoma of the lung
4. Grave's disease
5. Villous adenoma of the colon

Answer to Question 53 *is on page 255*

A 35-year-old schoolteacher has type I diabetes. She was diagnosed at the age of 21. She attends the diabetic follow-up clinic. Her glucose-monitoring diary shows that she has been having reasonable blood sugar measurements that are consistently between 5 and 7. Her last HBA1C was 7.5%. She has been otherwise well and has not changed her diet or daily routine significantly during the day. However, she has regularly been woken from sleep with hypoglycaemia and on one occasion required hospital attendance.

Her current insulin regimen is a short-acting insulin (Actrapid) tds before meals and an isophane (human Insulatard) preparation in the evening.

How would you recommend she adjusted her regimen?

1. Commence insulin glargine in place of her evening Insulatard dose
2. Commence rosiglitazone
3. Commence metformin
4. Increase her evening insulin Insulatard dose
5. Convert her to a twice-daily biphasic acting insulin preparation

Answer to Question 54 *is on page 256*

A 17-year-old Caucasian female RAF trainee presents with a 2-day history of jaundice. There were no preceding symptoms and her past health had always been good. She recently had her RAF medical and completed a course of vaccinations.

On examination she is markedly jaundiced, fully orientated and lucid. The abdomen is soft and non-tender with no organomegaly. There is evidence of peripheral oedema but no other stigmata of chronic liver disease. Blood pressure is 120/70 mmHg, pulse is 84/min regular, respiration rate is 14/min and temperature is 36.4°C.

INVESTIGATIONS

Hb	7.9 g/dL
MCV	100 fL
WCC	6.0×10^9/L
Platelets	40×10^9/L
Bilirubin	300 µmol/L
ALT	40 iu/L
ALP	30 iu/L
Albumin	22 g/dL
INR	4.5
APTT	40s
Sodium	134 mmol/L
Potassium	2.3 mmol/L
Urea	7.1 mmol/L
Creatinine	98 µmol/L
Bicarbonate	17 mmol/L
Cl-	113 mmol/L
Urine pH	5.0 (4.6–8.0)

In Type 1 RTA, urinary PH always more than 5.5 i.e. failure to acidify urine

a) The most likely diagnosis is:
   1. Chronic active hepatitis
   2. Wilson's disease
   3. Hereditary spherocytosis
   4. Paracetamol overdose
   5. Leptospirosis
   6. Haemachromatosis
   7. Salicylate overdose

b) Which of the following could account for her acidosis?
   1. Renal tubular acidosis type I (distal renal tubular acidosis)
   2. Lactic acidosis
   3. Salicylate overdose
   4. Diabetic ketoacidosis
   5. Renal tubular acidosis type II (proximal renal tubular acidosis)

A 30-year-old garage attendant is admitted with a 2-day history of vomiting. He has been short of breath for 4 weeks and has had a dry cough. On two occasions he has noticed some flecks of blood on his handkerchief. His urine has been dark on occasion and he has also noted that his ankles have become swollen. Previously well, he has smoked since he was 15.

On examination he is pale and hyperventilating. His blood pressure is 120/82 mmHg and he is apyrexial. Examination of the respiratory system reveals scattered crepitations throughout the lung fields. Urine dipstick protein ++, blood ++.

What is the most likely diagnosis?

1. Systemic lupus erythematosus
2. Wegener's granulomatosis
3. Legionaire's disease
4. Buerger's disease (thromboangiitis obliterans)
5. Goodpasture's syndrome (anti-GBM disease)

Answer to Question 56 *is on page 259*

A 50-year-old female with type II diabetes presents with intermittent numbness, tingling and burning pain in the radial digits of both hands. She has had the symptoms for 3 months and they awaken her at night, following which she cannot get back to sleep because she has a headache.

On examination there is no atrophy of her thenar muscles, but her hands appear large. Sensation to light touch is intact. Her reflexes are normal. Proximal muscle weakness is noted. Her observations are pulse 80/min regular, blood pressure 180/80 mmHg, and she is apyrexial. A urine dip is negative and a finger prick glucose test measures 6.2.

Which of the following would you next routinely perform?

1. Visual perimetry
2. Thyroid function tests
3. Cervical MRI scan
4. Serum insulin-like growth factor-1
5. Oral glucose tolerance test

A 58-year-old male with epilepsy is admitted through casualty having been found unconscious at home by his wife. He has been on various anti-epileptics. He is currently on sodium valproate. The following results are obtained 24 h later:

Sodium	135 mmol/L
Potassium	6.7 mmol/L
Urea	18 mmol/L
Creatinine	630 µmol/L
Calcium	1.84 mmol/L
Aspartate aminotransferase	86 iu/L
γ -GT	70 iu/L
Urine dipstick	blood ++
Ammonium sulphate test	coloured supernatant

a) What condition do these results suggest?
  1. Hepatorenal syndrome
  2. Pancreatitis
  3. Sodium valproate toxicity
  4. Rhabdomyolysis
  5. Obstructive renal failure secondary to an enlarged prostate

b) Suggest the cause in this patient:
  1. Myocardial infarction
  2. Status epilepticus
  3. Sepsis
  4. Drug toxicity
  5. Hypothermia

Answer to Question 58 *is on page 265*

A 42-year-old female has had severe Raynauds phenomenon. She went on to develop swelling of the fingers and feels constantly tired. She now presents with severe breathlessness and burning retrosternal discomfort.

On examination she: is breathless; has skin thickening of her hands, face and trunk; her peripheral joints are tender and painful; and she has bilateral basal crepitations. Her blood pressure is 160/90 mmHg.

Which of the following antibodies is associated with the clinical presentation?

1. Anti-neutrophil cytoplasmic antibody
2. Scl-70 antibody
3. Ro antibody
4. Anticentromere antibody
5. Jo-1 antibody

Answer to Question 59 *is on page 266*

A 13-year-old female underwent cardiac catheterization. Her parents had noticed that she was becoming increasingly breathless and blue.

	Saturation O_2(%)	Pressure (mmHg)
RA	74	26 mean
RV	76	110/5–10
PA	76	110/30
LV	92	105/0–10
Aorta	99	120/75

a) What is the diagnosis?
   1. Atrial septal defect
   2. Primary pulmonary hypertension
   3. Ventricular septal defect with a left-to-right shunt
   4. Ventricular septal defect with a right-to-left shunt
   5. Coarctation

b) What is the associated valvular abnormality?
   1. Aortic stenosis
   2. Aortic regurgitation
   3. Pulmonary stenosis
   4. Pulmonary regurgitation
   5. Mitral stenosis

Answer to Question 60 *is on page 268*

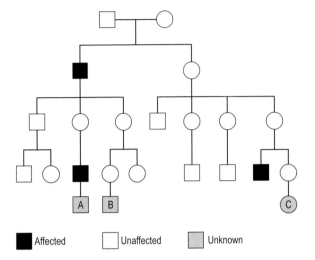

Affected   Unaffected   Unknown

a) In what Mendelian manner is this genetic trait transmitted?
   1. Autosomal recessive
   2. X-linked recessive
   3. Autosomal dominant
   4. X-linked dominant
   5. Anticipation

b) Assuming penetrance is complete and that none of the family marries another carrier or affected individual, what is the risk of patients A, B, and C being affected?

Patient A
   1. Not affected
   2. 1:2
   3. 1:4
   4. 1:8

Patient B
   1. Not affected
   2. 1:2
   3. 1:4
   4. 1:8

Patient C
   1. Not affected
   2. 1:2
   3. 1:4
   4. 1:8

Answer to Question 61 *is on page 269*

The following results are obtained in a 32-year-old female with galactorrhoea:

Sodium	136 mmol/L
Potassium	5.5 mmol/L
Bicarbonate	18 mmol/L
Calcium (corrected)	2.04 mmol/L
Hb	8.6 g/dL
MCV	92 fL
MCH	32 pg
TSH	2.4 mU/L

What is this woman's primary condition?

1. Primary hypothyroidism
2. Primary hypoparathyroidism
3. Prolactinoma
4. Chronic renal failure
5. Hypopituitarism

Answer to Question 62 *is on page 270*

A 71-year-old female has a 9-month history of dull aching in both calves after moderate exercise that settles with 5 min rest or with sitting down and stooping forward. Sphincter function has been normal but she has developed symmetrically numb thighs. Previously she has taken a variety of analgesics for low back pain. She has been a life-long smoker and has chronic obstructive airways disease. She takes inhalers intermittently and is not on regular medication.

On examination there is loss of her lumbar lordosis associated with reduced flexion and extension. Cranial nerves and the upper limb examination are normal. In the lower limbs, tone power and coordination are normal; the reflexes are symmetrical but reduced compared to the upper limbs. The plantar responses are flexor. Soft touch and pinprick sensation are reduced from below the groin to just above the knees laterally. Proprioception and vibration sense are normal. The femoral, popliteal, posterior tibial and dorsalis anterior arterial pulses are present both at rest and after exercise.

INVESTIGATIONS

Hb	14 g/dL
WBC	7.5×10^9/L
Platelets	455×10^9/L
Sodium	141 mmol/L
Potassium	3.9 mmol/L
Urea	7 mmol/L
Albumin	40 g/L
Calcium	2.3 mmol/L
Bilirubin	8 μmol/L
Aspartate transaminase	29 iu/L
Alkaline phosphatase	90 iu/L
IgG	15.5 g/L
IgA	2.2 g/L
IgM	3.0 g/L
Protein electrophoresis	normal
Bence-Jones protein	negative
CRP	5 mg/L
Chest X-ray	consistent with mild obstructive airways disease
Lumbar spine X-ray	lumbar spondylosis with marked osteophyte formation

Question continued overpage

a) What further investigation would you do to confirm the diagnosis?
1. Lower limb arterial dopplers before and after exercise
2. Isotope bone scan
3. Thyroid function tests
4. MRI lumbar spine
5. CPK

b) What is the diagnosis?
1. Peripheral vascular disease
2. Myopathy
3. McArdle's disease
4. Paget's disease of lumbar spine
5. Lumbar canal stenosis

Answer to Question 63 *is on page 271*

A 45-year-old mentally subnormal female presents in casualty with a broken arm after repeated falls. She has had epilepsy since childhood. Her last witnessed fit was 2 weeks before admission; prior to this she had been fit-free for 2 years. Pulmonary tuberculosis had been diagnosed 6 months previously. Her medication consists of phenytoin 400 mg, primidone 200 mg and Rifinah (combined rifampicin and isoniazid) 2 tablets daily.

Examination confirms the fracture. In addition she has mild nystagmus and ataxia. Otherwise physical examination is normal.

INVESTIGATIONS

Hb	11 g/L
MCV	105 fL
WBC	8×10^9/L – normal differential
Platelets	400×10^9/L
Sodium	136 mmol/L
Potassium	4.0 mmol/L
Urea	5 mmol/L
Albumin	40 g/L
Calcium	2.01 mmol/L
Phosphate	0.7 mmol/L
Bilirubin	6 μmol/L
Aspartate transaminase	28 iu/L
Alkaline phosphatase	180 iu/L

a) What is the diagnosis?
   1. Cerebellar space-occupying lesion
   2. Hypothyroidism
   3. Cerebellar abscess
   4. Phenytoin toxicity
   5. Rifampicin toxicity

b) What investigation would confirm the diagnosis?
   1. Blood cultures
   2. CT brain
   3. CSF examination
   4. Phenytoin levels
   5. Vitamin D level

Answer to Question 64 *is on page 272*

A 38-year-old female is admitted to hospital with a chest infection. On routine examination she is found to have abnormal pupillary reflexes.

	Direct light reaction	Consensual light reaction
Right pupil	Sluggish reaction	Normal
Left pupil	Normal	Sluggish

The right pupil reacts slowly to accommodation.

a) What abnormality is consistent with these findings?
1. Right optic neuritis
2. Left optic glioma
3. Right Holmes-Adie pupil
4. Right Argyll-Robertson pupil
5. Left optic neuritis

b) What other physical findings may be found?
1. Café-au-lait spots
2. Perphieral neuropathy
3. Shagreen macules
4. Diminished reflexes
5. Third nerve palsy

c) What is the underlying diagnosis?
1. Neurofibromatosis type I
2. Neurosyphilis
3. Multiple sclerosis
4. Idiopathic
5. Diabetes mellitis

Answer to Question 65 *is on page 273*

A 26-year-old solicitor undergoes a private 'health screen' before taking up a new job. The screening involves a range of blood tests, subsequent to which referral to the medical outpatient department is recommended. In the referral letter to the clinic, the following results are available:

Calcium	2.95 mmol/L
Serum magnesium	1.02 mmol/L
Phosphate	1.3 mmol/L
24-h urinary calcium excretion	2.1 mmol (normal range 2.5–7.5 mmol/24 h)

The patient is entirely well, but tells you that his mother had an operation on her neck in middle age because she was noted to have high blood calcium.

a) What is the likely diagnosis?
  1. Primary hyperparathyroidism
  2. Tertiary hyperparathyroidism
  3. Ectopic parathyroid hormone secretion
  4. Familial hypocalcuric hypercalcaemia
  5. Bony metastases

b) How would you manage this patient?
  1. Low calcium diet
  2. Intravenous pamidronate
  3. Parathyroid surgery
  4. No treatment required
  5. Furosemide

A 25-year-old female presents with acute renal failure. Diffuse interstitial shadowing is noted on chest X-ray and she has marked arterial hypoxaemia. Pulmonary function tests are as follows: FVC 67%, FEV1/VC 114%, DLCO 173%, KCO 275%, VA 62%.

a) What pathological process is occurring?
1. Active alveolitis
2. Alveolar haemorrhage
3. Pulmonary embolism
4. Pulmonary oedema
5. Interstitial pneumonitis

b) The most likely diagnosis is:
1. Acute asthma
2. *Pneumocystis carinii* pneumonia
3. Microscopic polyangiitis
4. Drug induced
5. Atypical pneumonia

A 37-year-old trout farmer presents with a 7-day history of fever, myalgias, nausea and severe frontal headache. He has experienced occasional colicky abdominal pain and has vomited in casualty. On two occasions he has noticed haematuria. One month previously he returned from his honeymoon in France but has not otherwise travelled abroad. At the age of 6 he suffered an episode of infectious hepatitis and there is a family history of diabetes mellitus. He drinks 5 pints of beer most evenings but does not smoke. He takes paracetamol occasionally for long-standing lower back pain.

On examination he is pyrexial, has a temperature of 38.5°C and is icteric. Bilateral subconjunctival suffusion and a purpuric rash over both calves are noted. There is no asterixis and he is alert. He has marked photophobia but no neck stiffness. In the abdomen he has smooth 4-cm hepatomegaly.

INVESTIGATIONS

Hb	11.3 g/dL
WBC	15.9×10^9/L – 90% neutrophils
Platelets	118×10^9/L
Sodium	132 mmol/L
Potassium	4.5 mmol/L
Urea	27.8 mmol/L
Creatinine	305 µmol/L
Bilirubin	76 µmol/L
Aspartate aminotransferase	78 iu/L
Alkaline phosphatase	642 iu/L
PT	13 s
APTT	32 s
Urine dipstick	protein ++, blood ++
Urine microscopy	occasional white cells, occasional red cells, no casts

a) What is the most likely diagnosis?
1. Acute hepatitis A
2. Infectious mononucleosis
3. Leptospirosis
4. Legionella pneumonia
5. Malaria

b) What treatment would you recommend?
1. Oral doxycycline
2. IV benzylpenicillin
3. Ribavirin
4. IV quinine
5. Oral erythromycin and rifampicin

Answer to Question 68 *is on page 276*

This is the ECG of a 14-year-old male with recurrent dizzy spells.

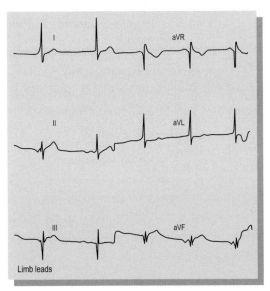

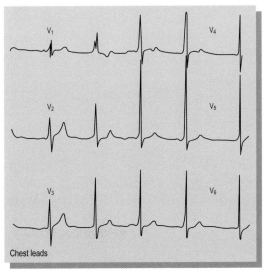

What is the diagnosis?

1. Wolff-Parkinson-White syndrome
2. Romano Ward syndrome
3. Hypertrophic cardiomyopathy
4. Atrial septal defect
5. Trifasicular block

A 35-year-old male diagnosed with HIV was commenced on highly active anti-retroviral therapy (HAART). He had not previously been on any treatment. At week 8 of therapy his viral load was 10 000 copies/mL and his CD4 count was 350 cells/μL.

Which of the following is correct?

1. Treatment was likely to have commenced because his CD4 count was above 350 cells/μL
2. It is most likely that he is poorly compliant with treatment
3. Primary prophylaxis for an opportunist infection is required
4. A resistance assay is not currently indicated
5. Lipodystrophy does not complicate protease inhibitor based regimens

Answer to Question 70 *is on page 278*

A 22-year-old female is 3 months post-renal transplantation. She presents to the clinic with diarrhoea and a fever. She also complains of a burning retrosternal discomfort when eating. She is currently maintained on prednisolone, azathioprine and ciclosporin.

Her blood results show mildly raised transaminases.

What is the most likely diagnosis?

1. Cryptosporidium infection
2. Azathioprine toxicity
3. Cytomegalovirus infection
4. Ciclosporin toxicity
5. Bacterial overgrowth

The following results are obtained in a 32-year-old female with a blood pressure of 184/114 mmHg.

INVESTIGATIONS

Sodium	135 mmol/L
Potassium	5.2 mmol/L
Urea	11.2 mmol/L
Creatinine	212 µmol/L
Albumin	30 g/L
Urinalysis	blood non-haemolyzed trace
Protein	5.4 g/24 h
Urine microscopy	scanty red cells and granular casts
HbA1c	3.4%
ANA	1:320 speckled pattern
Renal biopsy	immunofluorescence: linear IgG on glomerular basement membrane

a) What is the diagnosis?
   1. Diabetic nephropathy
   2. Hypertensive nephropathy
   3. Systemic lupus erythematosus
   4. Polyarteritis nodosa
   5. Goodpastures' disease

b) What histological pattern is likely to present in the kidney?
   1. Minimal change glomerulonephritis
   2. Glomerosclerosis
   3. Membraneous nephritis
   4. Mesangio-proliferative nephritis
   5. Cresentic glomerular nephritis

Answer to Question 72 *is on page 280*

A 60-year-old female was brought to casualty unconscious. Her blood glucose was 2.1 mmol/L. She was resuscitated with intravenous glucose. She gave a 3-month history of early morning dizziness but otherwise her past history was unremarkable. The following investigations were performed:

Fasting blood glucose	2.2 mmol/L
Blood insulin	16 mU/L
Hb	14 g/dL
MCV	84 fL
Urea/electrolytes/liver function tests	normal
C-peptide levels	high

a) What is the cause of her hypoglycaemia?
  1. Ethanol
  2. Insulinoma
  3. Pituitary insufficiency
  4. Exogenous insulin administration
  5. Adrenal failure

b) What further test will help to confirm the diagnosis?
  1. Anti-insulin receptor antibodies
  2. Serum cortisol levels
  3. CT scan of pancreas
  4. Ethanol levels
  5. MRI head

A 12-year-old male is referred to outpatients with nocturnal enuresis. His mother comments that he is easily tired by sport and is not doing well at school. He is normotensive and on the 8th centile for height.

INVESTIGATIONS

Sodium	145 mmol/L
Potassium	2.8 mmol/L
Bicarbonate	35 mmol/L
Chloride	80 mmol/L
Urea	5 mmol/L
Glucose	4.4 mmol/L
24-h urine	60 mmol of potassium, 60 mmol of sodium

What is the diagnosis?

1. Conn's syndrome
2. Hypokalaemic periodic paralysis
3. Bartter's syndrome
4. Villous adenoma
5. Renal tubular acidosis

Answer to Question 74 *is on page 282*

A 17-year-old female has a syncopal episode while playing football. Her mother says that she has always been fit and well but had been started on erythromycin for an ear infection 2 days previously.

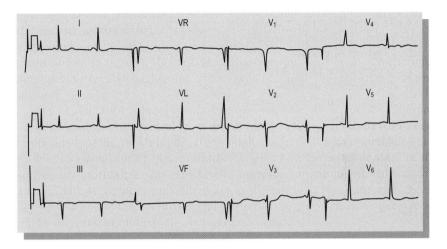

Which of the following abnormalities is the most relevant?

1. Voltage criteria for left ventricular hypertrophy
2. Inverted T waves in leads V1–V3
3. Presence of U waves
4. Abnormal PR interval
5. Prolonged QT interval

A 29-year-old female presents to the clinic with a short history of headaches that are worse in the morning, and double vision. On examination, the patient weighs 102 kg, there is papilloedema, and a partial right VI nerve palsy, but no other abnormal neurological signs.

a) What is the most likely diagnosis?
  1. Subarachnoid haemorrhage
  2. Classical migraine
  3. Benign intracranial hypertension
  4. Intracerebral tumour
  5. Saggital sinus thrombosis

b) Which of the following would be the most appropriate treatment?
  1. Radiotherapy
  2. Sumatriptan
  3. Anticoagulation
  4. Diuretics
  5. Ergotamine

Answer to Question 76 *is on page 285*

A 45-year-old male presents with fatigue, lethargy and swollen ankles, which had been noted over the previous 6 months. He is an intravenous drug user and is known to be hepatitis C positive. Four years previously, he was admitted with infected sores secondary to drug injection and a diagnosis of osteomyelitis of the right femur was made. He was treated for 3 months with IV antibiotics, underwent surgery and had a medullary nail inserted but was left with a discharging sinus.

On examination he is found to be alert, orientated and apyrexial. He has been wheelchair bound following surgery to his right leg. The presence of peripheral oedema is confirmed. There is no evidence of a rash. A urine dip reveals proteinuria +++. (Review of the notes shows that a urine dip performed a year previously was also positive for protein.)

His electrolytes show deranged renal function. A renal ultrasound reveals no evidence of obstruction or thrombus, and isoechoeic kidneys which measure 10.0 cm on the left and 10.5 cm on the right.

What is the most likely renal pathology?

1. Membranous glomerulonephritis
2. Focal segmental glomerulonephritis
3. Minimal change disease
4. Renal amyloidosis
5. Cryoglobulinaemia

A 40-year-old female presents to the clinic concerned that she may have polycystic kidney disease. She has heard that this is an inherited disorder and her aunt may have had 'cysts on her kidney' and died unexpectedly aged 41.

What would be the best method to exclude the diagnosis?

1. Ultrasound abdomen
2. CT abdomen
3. Gene studies
4. MR angiogram
5. Urine dipstick

Question 79

A 55-year-old male presents with a 12-hour history of severe abdominal pain and vomiting. He had been recently commenced on a thiazide diuretic for high blood pressure. On examination he is unwell, sweaty and tachycardic, with a blood pressure of 115/85 mmHg. His abdomen is diffusely tender and bowel sounds are absent.

INVESTIGATIONS

Hb	13 g/dL
WBC	14×10^9/L
Platelets	245×10^9/L
Sodium	143 mmol/L
Potassium	3.9 mmol/L
Urea	9 mmol/L
Albumin	27 g/L
Calcium	1.9 mmol/L
Phosphate	0.8 mmol/L
Bilirubin	25 µmol/L
Aspartate transaminase	40 iu/L
Glucose	13 mmol/L
pO_2	8.8 kPa
pCO_2	4.0 kPa

a) What is the likely diagnosis?
   1. Acute intermittent porphyria
   2. Acute appendicitis
   3. Acute bowel perforation
   4. Acute pancreatitis
   5. Acute pulmonary embolism

b) How would you confirm your diagnosis?
   1. Erect chest X-ray
   2. Serum amylase
   3. V/Q scan
   4. Laparotomy
   5. Lead levels
   6. Measure serum delta-aminolaevulinic acid
   7. CRP

Answer to Question 79 *is on page 288*

A 33-year-old female was found to have a murmur on a routine medical examination. She denied any symptoms.

The results of cardiac catheterization show:

	Saturation O_2 %	Pressure
RA	70	mean 4
RV	71	30/3
PA	80	30/15
PCWP		12

a) What is the diagnosis?
   1. pulmonary stenosis
   2. patent ductus arteriosis
   3. mitral stenosis
   4. atrial septal defect
   5. ventricular septal defect

b) What is the treatment?
   1. Valvotomy
   2. Valve replacement
   3. Surgical correction
   4. Angiographic embolization
   5. Prostaglandin antagonists

A 38-year-old Caucasian female presents with a 2-day history of a painful, swollen right leg. Eight years previously she had a similar episode, which spontaneously resolved. Three weeks previously she had had an upper respiratory tract infection for which her family doctor prescribed amoxicillin. Over the previous 3 years she had noticed the occasional passing of dark urine, particularly first thing in the morning. She has also had some colicky abdominal pain. Her father died at the age of 50 from a cerebrovascular accident and there is a strong family history of hypertension. She smokes 20 cigarettes a day, drinks no alcohol and is on no regular medication.

On examination she is pyrexial with a temperature of 38.2°C, is normotensive and has a tense, erythematous, painful, swollen left calf.

INVESTIGATIONS

Hb	8.9 g/dL
WBC	2.3×10^9/L (40% neutrophils)
Platelets	43×10^9/L
Sodium	143 mmol/L
Potassium	3.6 mmol/L
Urea	4.3 mmol/L
Bilirubin	12 μmol/L
Aspartate aminotransferase	32 iu/L
Alkaline phosphatase	124 iu/L
PT	12 s
APTT	37 s
Fibrinogen	2.6 g/L
Thrombin time	15 s

a) Which of the following would account for her presentation?
  1. Acute intermittent porphyria
  2. Paroxysmal nocturnal haemoglobinuria
  3. Alkaptonuria
  4. Sickle cell crisis
  5. Behçet syndrome

b) How would you confirm your underlying diagnosis?
  1. Right leg venogram
  2. Haemoglobin electrophoresis
  3. Blood film
  4. Ham's test
  5. Coomb's test

Answer to Question 81 *is on page 290*

A 34-year-old male presents with a 1-week history of pain in the left eye, which is worse on movement associated with blurred vision. One year previously, he had noticed that his ability to play tennis had been transiently impaired by apparent weakness of his right foot, but he had not sought medical advice as the symptoms had resolved after about a month. He had, however, been treated by his GP for acute labyrinthitis about 3 months before developing his current problem.

a) What is the likely diagnosis?
  1. Cerebrovascular disease and multiple transient ischaemic attacks
  2. Motor neuron disease
  3. Multiple sclerosis
  4. Cerebral vasculitis
  5. Vitamin B_{12} deficiency

b) What sign is most likely to be present on opthalmological assessment?
  1. Reduced colour vision
  2. Homonomous hemianopia
  3. Optic atrophy
  4. Bitemporal hemianopia
  5. Ptosis

c) Which of the following investigations would you next perform?
  1. Echocardiogram
  2. 24-h electrocardiogram
  3. Magnetic resonance imaging of the head and spinal cord
  4. Computed tomography of the head
  5. Schilling test

Answer to Question 82 *is on page 291*

A 65-year-old male is admitted through casualty with marked shortness of breath. On examination he is in atrial fibrillation with a radial rate of 145 and an apical-radial deficit of 30, and has blood pressure of 148/92 mmHg, jugular venous pressure is elevated at 8 cm, cardiomegaly, gallop rhythm and an apical pansystolic murmur are present. Both lung bases are dull to percussion and there are end-inspiratory crepitations to the mid zones. Gross pitting ankle oedema to the mid thighs is present. On admission he is taking no regular medication.

INVESTIGATIONS

Sodium	128 mmol/L
Potassium	2.9 mmol/L
Bicarbonate	30 mmol/L
Urea	8 mmol/L
Albumin	24 g/L
Bilirubin	43 μmol/L
Alkaline phosphatase	601 iu/L
Aspartate aminotransferase	40 iu/L
γ -GT	50 iu/L
Chest X-ray	upper lobe blood diversion, alveolar oedema and bilateral effusions
Urine dipstick	trace of protein

What is the diagnosis?

1. Nephrotic syndrome
2. Chronic liver disease
3. Congestive cardiac failure
4. Protein-losing enteropathy
5. Cushing's syndrome

Answer to Question 83 *is on page 292*

A 41-year-old female was admitted with an upper gastrointestinal tract haemorrhage. She complained of mild upper abdominal pain for 1 year; otherwise she was well. She was not on regular medication. She was unmarried, worked as a journalist; smoked 20 cigarettes per day and on average drank 2 glasses of wine per week.

On examination she was well tanned but had pale mucous membranes. There were two spider naevi on her upper trunk but no palmar erythema, jaundice or lymphadenopathy. Examination of the heart and lungs was normal. On palpation of her abdomen her liver was one finger-breadth below the costal margin and the tip of her spleen could be felt. Neurological examination was normal.

INVESTIGATIONS

Hb	12.5 g/dL
WBC	5.5 × 10⁹/L
Platelets	200 × 10⁹/L
MCV	88 fL
ESR	40 mm in the first hour
Sodium	135 mmol/L
Potassium	4 mmol/L
Urea	5 mmol/L
Albumin	35 g/L
IgG	16 g/L (5.3–16.5)
IgM	9 g/L (0.5–2.0)
IgA	2 g/L (0.8–4)
Calcium	1.9 mmol/L
Phosphate	0.6 mmol/L
Glucose	5.0 mmol/L
Bilirubin	12 μmol/L
Aspartate transaminase	30 iu/L
Alkaline phosphatase	300 iu/L
γ -GT	80 iu/L
Prothrombin time	12 s
Chest X-ray	normal
Abdominal X-ray	normal
Urinalysis	normal

Give the most likely underlying diagnosis?

1. Wilson's disease
2. Autoimmune hepatitis
3. Primary biliary cirrhosis
4. Alcoholic liver disease
5. Haemochromatosis

Question 85

A 7-year-old male is admitted following a grand mal convulsion. On examination he is on the 25th centile for height and weight. He has short 4th and 5th metacarpals. Trousseau and Chvostek signs are positive. There is evidence of intellectual impairment.

Glucose	4 mmol/L
Calcium	1.7 mmol/L
Albumin	39 g/L
Phosphate	1.9 mmol/L
Alkaline phosphatase	190 iu/L
Urea	4 mmol/L
Creatinine	75 µmol/L
Hb	11 g/dL

a) What is the cause of his convulsion?
   1. Hypophosphataemic rickets
   2. Primary hypoparathyroidism
   3. Hereditary vitamin D resistant rickets
   4. Pseudohypoparathyroidism
   5. Pseudopseudohypoparathyroidism

b) How would you confirm the diagnosis?
   1. 24-h urinary calcium
   2. Calcitonin levels
   3. Serum albumin
   4. Isotope scan of parathyroid glands
   5. Infusion of PTH with measurement of urinary phosphate and cyclic AMP

Answer to Question 85 *is on page 295*

Question 86

A 52-year-old female is admitted to casualty feeling unwell. She has a severe headache, which came on suddenly while she was watching television, and has vomited once. She is apyrexial, but has some neck stiffness and is drowsy. Her pulse is 100/min sinus rhythm and blood pressure 150/95 mmHg. She has no other focal neurological signs, and fundoscopy is normal.

a) What is the most likely diagnosis?
  1. Acute meningitis
  2. Acute labyrinthitis
  3. Migraine
  4. Subarachnoid haemorrhage
  5. Ischaemic stroke

b) What is the most important initial investigation that is required?
  1. Echocardiogram
  2. CT scan of head
  3. Lumbar puncture
  4. Renal ultrasound
  5. X-ray of neck

c) What is the commonest cause of this problem?
  1. Bacterial sepsis
  2. Viral sepsis
  3. Iatrogenic – warfarin
  4. Intracranial aneurysm
  5. Tachyarrthymias

d) What treatment would you initiate?
  1. Nifedipine
  2. Nimodipine
  3. Dexamethasone
  4. IV broad spectrum antibiotics
  5. Aspirin

Answer to Question 86 *is on page 296*

A 26-year-old male smoker has become increasingly short of breath. He has not had any previous respiratory problems but as a child was always smaller then his peers.

Examination reveals hyperinflated lungs, and a palpable liver and splenic edge. His lung function tests are as following:

PEFR	220	Pred 550
FEV1	2.0	Pred 4
FVC	4	Pred 5.5
TLC	7	Pred 6.4
KCO	0.7	Pred 1.6

The chest X-ray shows hyperinflated lung fields with evidence of reduced vascularity at the bases.

a) What is the most likely diagnosis?
1. Cystic fibrosis
2. Alpha-1-antitrypsin deficiency
3. Kartagener's syndrome
4. Selective immunoglobulin deficiency
5. Gaucher's disease

b) How would you best confirm the diagnosis?
1. Sweat test
2. CT thorax
3. Immunoglobulin levels
4. Alpha-1-antitrypsin electrophoresis
5. Liver biopsy

Answer to Question 87 *is on page 298*

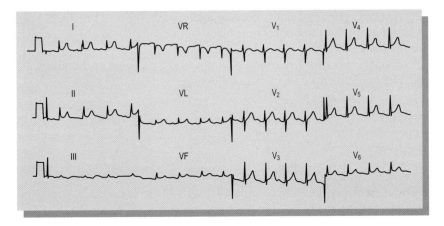

This ECG has been recorded from a 28-year-old male who has presented with severe central chest pain. He has no known risk factors for coronary artery disease.

Which of the following is least likely to account for his symptoms?

1. Post-cocaine use
2. Pericarditis
3. Normal variant
4. Acute coronary syndrome
5. Brugada syndrome

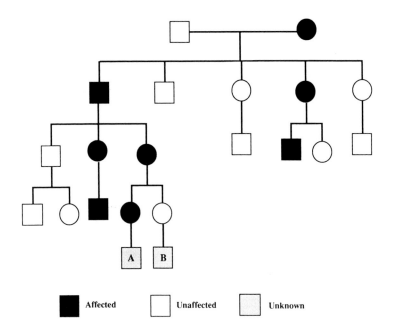

Affected **Unaffected** **Unknown**

The affected members in this family were below the 3rd centile in height and had a plasma phosphate consistently below 0.45 mmol/L; their alkaline phosphatase was between 150 and 200 iu/L and their calcium was within the normal range.

a) What is the diagnosis?
  1. Primary hypoparathyroidism
  2. Familial hypophosphataemic rickets
  3. Pseudopseudohypoparathyroidism
  4. Primary hyperparathyroidism
  5. Renal tubular acidosis

b) How is the defect inherited?
  1. X-linked recessive
  2. Autosomal dominant
  3. X-linked dominant
  4. Autosomal recessive
  5. Somatic mutation

c) What is the risk of A and B being affected?
  1. A nil, B 50%
  2. A 50%, B nil
  3. A 25%, B 25%
  4. A 50%, B 25%
  5. A nil, B 25%

Answer to Question 89 *is on page 301*

A 43-year-old female presents with a history of increasing tiredness. Seven years previously she was successfully treated with combined chemotherapy and radiotherapy for stage IV Hodgkin's disease.

INVESTIGATIONS

Hb	10.2 g/dL
WBC	3.4 × 10⁹/L, neutrophils 34%
Blood film	Pelger cells and occasional blasts
Platelets	49 × 10⁹/L
MCV	108 fL

What is the likely cause of her anaemia?

1. Vitamin B$_{12}$ deficiency
2. Hypothyroidism
3. Reoccurrence of lymphoma
4. Myelodysplasia
5. Acute myeloid leukaemia

Answer to Question 90 *is on page 302*

A 46-year-old female is brought into casualty, complaining of palpitations and breathlessness, but no chest pain. An ECG shows atrial fibrillation which resolves spontaneously. A chest X-ray shows cardiomegaly and pulmonary congestion.

The following results were obtained:

Haemoglobin	11 g/dL
WCC	4×10^9/L
MCV	102 fL
Platelets	110×10^9/L
ESR	25 mm/h

Echocardiography

LV end systolic volume	140 mL
LV end diastolic volume	170 mL
Ejection fraction	20%
Moderate mitral regurgitation	

a) What is the underlying diagnosis?
  1. Restrictive cardiomyopathy
  2. Dilated cardiomyopathy
  3. Hypertrophic obstructive cardiomyopathy
  4. Mixed mitral valve disease
  5. Acute rheumatic fever

b) What is the likely aetiology?
  1. Viral infection
  2. Alcohol abuse
  3. Streptococcal infection
  4. Endocardial fibrosis
  5. Congenital defect of mitral valve

Answer to Question 91 *is on page 303*

A 10-year-old male is admitted for investigation. His mother has noted that he has become progressively clumsy. On examination he is alert and orientated. Abnormal findings are a right-sided intention tremor and right-sided nystagmus.

INVESTIGATIONS

Hb	16 g/dL
WBC	6×10^9/L
Platelets	225×10^9/L
PCV	55%
Urea and electrolytes	normal

a) The history and signs point to a diagnosis in which part of the brain?
1. Left vestibular system
2. Left lobe of cerebellum
3. Basal ganglia
4. Right lobe of cerebellum
5. Right temporal lobe

b) Give one unifying diagnosis:
1. Friederich's ataxia
2. Refsum's disease
3. Medulloblastoma
4. Von Hippel-Lindau disease
5. Von Recklinghausen's disease

Question 93

The following data was acquired from cardiac catheterization of a 26-year-old man with episodic dizziness.

	Saturation O_2(%)	Pressure (mmHg)
RA	73	Mean 5
		A-wave 7
RV	75	97/0–10
PA	74	24/14
LV	96	130/0–10
Femoral artery	92	185/60

a) What is the most likely cause for the systemic desaturation?
   1. Coarctation of the aorta
   2. Atrial septal defect
   3. Ventricular septal defect
   4. Pulmonary hypertension
   5. Lung disease

b) What is the valve lesion?
   1. Aortic stenosis
   2. Pulmonary stenosis
   3. Pulmonary regurgitation
   4. Mitral stenosis
   5. Mitral regurgitation

c) Echocardiography shows a thickened right ventricle. What other abnormality do you suspect?
   1. Coartation of the aorta
   2. Aortic stenosis
   3. Pulmonary regurgitation
   4. Atrial septal defect
   5. Over-riding aorta

Answer to Question 93 *is on page 305*

A 12-year-old male developed recurrent upper abdominal pain and intermittent diarrhoea after returning from a short holiday to Leningrad with his school. The stools were bulky, pale and offensive. He had no fever and had an excellent appetite. In the past he had had whooping cough and since then had had regular attacks of bronchitis during the winter, but had been able to play games and had had little time off school.

On examination he has no rash, anaemia, clubbing, lymphadenopathy or jaundice. His height is on the 50th centile and his weight is 60% of that predicted for an average boy of his age. His two other siblings are both within the normal range. Examination of the cardiovascular system is normal. Examination of the chest reveals crackles at his left base and right mid-zone. On palpation his abdomen is soft and there is no organomegaly. His right colon is easily palpable and loaded with faeces. Examination of the CNS is normal.

INVESTIGATIONS

Hb	13 g/dL
WBC	9×10^9/L
Platelets	400×10^9/L
ESR	50 mm in the first hour
Sodium	137 mmol/L
Potassium	4.1 mmol/L
Urea	6 mmol/L
Albumin	25 g/L
Total protein	70 g/L
Vitamin B_{12}	300 ng/L
Folate	2 µg/L
Iron	17 µmol/L
TIBC	50 µmol/L
Faecal fat excretion	28 mmol/L

Chest X-ray shows small patches of atelectasis in the left base. Abdominal X-ray shows a dilated colon loaded with faeces.

a) What is the most likely diagnosis?
  1. Hypogammaglobulinaemia
  2. Coeliac disease
  3. Cystic fibrosis
  4. Kartagener's syndrome
  5. Giardiasis

Question continued overpage

b) Which two investigations would you request to help confirm your diagnosis?
  1. Colonoscopy
  2. Jejunal biopsy
  3. A sweat test
  4. Immunoglobulins
  5. Echocardiogram
  6. Stool culture

Answer to Question 94 *is on page 306*

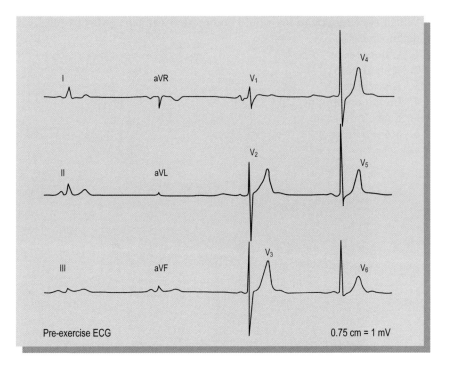

I aVR V1 V4

II aVL V2 V5

III aVF V3 V6

Pre-exercise ECG   0.75 cm = 1 mV

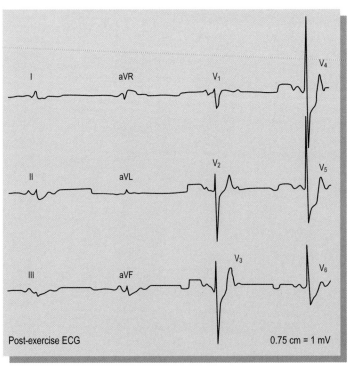

I aVR V1 V4

II aVL V2 V5

III aVF V3 V6

Post-exercise ECG   0.75 cm = 1 mV

Question on overpage

This is the tracing of an exercise tolerance test. Standard Bruce protocol was used. The test was terminated at 5 min 22 s with chest pain.

a) What is the most likely pathology underlying this change?
   1. Coronary artery disease of the right coronary artery
   2. Coronary artery disease of the left anterior descending artery
   3. Hypertrophic cardiomyopathy
   4. Coronary artery disease of the left circumflex artery
   5. Coronary artery disease of the posterior descending artery

b) The patient's resting blood pressure on no treatment is 110/70 mmHg. What other condition must be considered?
   1. Aortic regurgitation
   2. Mitral stenosis
   3. Mitral regurgitation
   4. Aortic stenosis
   5. Pulmonary stenosis

Answer to Question 95 *is on page 307*

A 35-year-old diagnosed with HIV in 2001 presents with a generalized rash, leg swelling and lymphadenopathy after a recent trip to Ibiza. Aside from his highly active retroviral therapeutic regimen he takes no other medication. Examination reveals a widespread pink maculopapular rash over the trunk, arms and hands, and axillary lymphadenopathy. Oral examination reveals painless mucosal ulceration. He also has pitting oedema present to the mid-shin.

A urine dipstick performed in the clinic shows proteinuria ++++.

a) What is the likely diagnosis?
  1. A drug reaction
  2. Secondary syphilis *(Treponema pallidum)*
  3. Hepatitis C
  4. Lymphoma
  5. Measles

Subsequent investigation also included a renal biopsy.

b) What is this likely to have shown?
  1. Membranous glomerulonephritis
  2. Minimal change glomerulonephritis
  3. Crescenteric glomerulonephritis
  4. Mesangial proliferative glomerulonephritis
  5. Interstitial nephritis

Answer to Question 96 *is on page 308*

A patient has severe aortic regurgitation but the echocardiogram shows well-preserved left ventricular function. She is awaiting assessment for surgery. She has no other history of cardiovascular disease and is a non-smoker. Her GP had commenced her on an angiotensin converting enzyme inhibitor (ACEI) 3 months previously to control her blood pressure and has written to say that the blood pressure has been consistently elevated.

On examination her pulse is 74/min regular and her blood pressure is 150/85 mmHg. On auscultation there is an early diastolic murmur heard loudest in the aortic area. There is an additional mid-diastolic murmur at the apex. The left ventricle is not displaced.

Which of the following options would you choose?

1. Commence nifedipine
2. Start a beta blocker
3. Start low dose digoxin
4. Start diltiazem
5. Monitor blood pressure and review in 3 months

Answer to Question 97 *is on page 311*

A 20-year-old female presented to the outpatient department complaining of recurrent generalized itching and shortness of breath. In recent months she had had three episodes of pleurisy and mild shortness of breath on exertion. Her friends had commented to her that her holiday tan had lasted well into the winter. In the past she had experienced mild Raynaud's phenomenon which had required no treatment. She worked in an office and was not exposed to industrial dusts or chemicals. She took no regular medication and was a non-smoker. Her two maternal aunts had rheumatoid arthritis.

Examination revealed a fit-looking, young woman who was well tanned. The skin on her forearms and fingers was boggy and oedematous but there was no desquamation. She had no lymphadenopathy, cyanosis, anaemia, clubbing or clinical jaundice. Her pulse was 80/min regular, blood pressure 150/90 mmHg, and the jugular venous pressure was visible 1 cm above the angle of Louis. Her heart sounds were normal, apart from a loud P2 and there were several fine bilateral crackles heard at both lung bases.

INVESTIGATIONS

Hb	13 g/dL
ESR	20 mm in first hour
CRP	10 mg/L
Urea	4.6 mmol/L
Creatinine	145 µmol/L
AST	60 iu/L
ALT	58 iu/L
Bilirubin	10 umol/L
Alkaline phosphatase	180 iu/L
Rheumatoid factor	negative
Antinuclear antibody	1/80 homogeneous
Complement profile	normal
Serum angiotensin-converting enzyme	normal
Chest X-ray	bilateral fine linear shadowing/ atelectasis
Ventilation/perfusion scan	normal
Lung function tests	
FEV1	2.0 L
VC	2.4 L
PEFR	5.5 L/s
TLC	3.0 L
TLCO	80% predicted
VA	1.8 L (70%)
KCO	90% predicted

Question continued overpage

a) What is the most likely diagnosis?
 1. Systemic lupus erythematosus
 2. Primary biliary cirrhosis
 3. Systemic sclerosis
 4. Primary haemachromatosis
 5. Cryptogenic fibrosing alveolitis

b) What complications have occurred? Name three:
 1. Interstitial pneumonitis
 2. Congestive cardiac failure
 3. Pulmonary hypertension
 4. Glomerulonephritis
 5. Acute hepatitis
 6. Renovascular disease

Answer to Question 98 *is on page 312*

A 75-year-old male presents with tiredness. On examination he is pale, and has widespread lymphadenopathy and a 6-cm spleen.

INVESTIGATIONS

Hb	7.6 g/dL
WBC	28×10^9/L – 92% lymphocytes
Platelets	52×10^9/L
Blood film	polychromasia and spherocytes
Reticulocytes	8%
Serum haptoglobins	undetected

a) What is the likely diagnosis?
   1. Hereditary spherocytosis
   2. Acute myeloid leukaemia with autoimmune haemolytic anaemia
   3. Chronic lymphatic leukaemia with autoimmune haemolytic anaemia
   4. Myelodysplasia
   5. Chronic myeloid leukaemia

b) How would you confirm your diagnosis?
   1. Indirect Coombs' test
   2. Bone marrow
   3. Direct Coombs' test
   4. CT chest and abdomen
   5. Ham's lysis test

Answer to Question 99 *is on page 313*

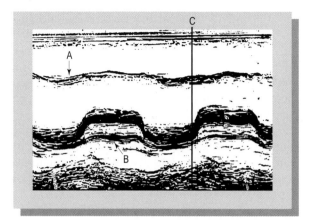

This is the M-mode echocardiogram of a 40-year-old female.

a) What valve lesion is present?
1. Aortic stenosis
2. Mitral regurgitation
3. Mitral stenosis
4. Tricuspid stenosis
5. Tricuspid regurgitation

b) What is structure B?
1. Posterior leaflet aortic valve
2. Anterior leaflet mitral valve
3. Anterior leaflet tricuspid valve
4. Posterior leaflet mitral valve
5. Left ventricle

c) What physical sign would coincide with line C?
1. 1st heart sound
2. 2nd heart sound
3. Systolic murmur
4. Opening snap
5. Diastolic murmur

Answer to Question 100 *is on page 314*

A 26-year-old female attends the outpatient department with a 2-month history of left hip pain – worse on weight-bearing and on exertion. Some relief is obtained from ibuprofen. She has a complex previous medical history: 18 months previously she underwent a trans-sphenoidal hypophysectomy for a benign pituitary lesion, which has resulted in pituitary failure. She had been on thyroid replacement therapy with 150 μg T4 for 2 years, and oestrogen therapy for 9 months. Perioperatively she had received 4 mg 6-hourly of dexamethasone for 3 weeks, and had been taking 2 mg 12-hourly for the last 12 months. On examination her weight is 102 kg and her height is 5ft 1 inch. She is apyrexial. Chest cardiovascular and abdominal examinations are normal. There is marked restriction of external and internal rotation of the left hip, with groin pain. FBC and ESR normal.

a) What is the most likely explanation for her hip pain?
1. Osteoarthritis secondary to excess weight
2. Osteoporotic fracture of femur
3. Septic arthritis
4. Avascular necrosis of femoral head
5. Trochanteric bursitis

b) What is the next appropriate investigation?
1. DEXA scan
2. Isotope bone scan
3. Plain X-ray of the hips
4. Magnetic resonance image of the hip
5. Ultrasound scan of the hip

Answer to Question 101 *is on page 315*

Question 102

A 35-year-old female is admitted confused, pyrexial and vomiting. Her flatmate reports that she has been unwell for the last 3 months and has lost weight. Three days previously she was bed-bound with a severe cold. Her brother, who was called urgently by the flatmate, collapsed in casualty, and was found to be hypoglycaemic. He responded to intravenous dextrose; it transpired that he had missed his evening meal in his rush to visit his sister. He has been insulin-dependent for 5 years.

On examination the sister is disorientated in time and place; her temperature is 39°C, her pulse 110/min irregularly irregular and her blood pressure is 100/60 mmHg. There is no neck stiffness and no focal neurological signs. The emergency team has performed a CT head scan and this has been reported as normal. The duty SHO has performed a lumbar puncture and the following results are available:

INVESTIGATIONS

Hb	14 g/dL
WBC	9×10^9/L–70% neutrophils
Sodium	140 mmol/L
Potassium	4 mmol/L
Urea	13 mmol/L
Albumin	35 g/L
Calcium	2.6 mmol/L
Phosphate	1.2 mmol/L
Glucose	5.2 mmol/L
CSF	opening pressure 9 cm/CSF
Protein	0.45 g/L
Glucose	4 mmol/L
Cell count	3 lymphocytes/mm^3

a) What is the likely diagnosis?
   1. Acute viral gastroenteritis
   2. Viral meningitis
   3. Acute thyrotoxicosis
   4. Adrenal crisis
   3. Acute urinary tract infection

b) How would you treat the patient? Name two treatments:
   1. IV hydrocortisone and fludrocortisone
   2. IV antibiotics
   3. IV carbimazole
   4. IV beta blocker
   5. IV thyroxine

Answer to Question 102 *is on page 316*

Investigations for a 5-year-old child:

PT	14 s	(15–19)
APPT	80 s	(30–46)
TT	12 s	(15–19)
Fibrinogen	3.5 g	(2–4)
Bleeding time	5 min	(3–9)
Normal platelet function		

a) What is the likely diagnosis?
   1. Disseminated intravascular coagulation
   2. Haemophilia A
   3. Haemophilia B
   4. Lupus anticoagulant
   5. Von-Willebrand's disease

b) What are the likely complications? Name two:
   1. Increased thrombosis
   2. Prolonged bleeding
   3. Recurrent haemarthroses
   4. Spontaneous bruising
   5. Disseminated intravascular coagulation

Answer to Question 103 *is on page 317*

An 86-year-old patient attends clinic with some increased breathlessness on mild exertion not associated with chest pain. He is known to have severe aortic stenosis (peak valve gradient 60 mmHg). He has declined surgery. He still remains active and does his own shopping. His current medication is aspirin 75 mg.

Examination is consistent with aortic stenosis: his apex is slightly displaced and there are some crepitations in both lung bases. His jugular venous pressure is not raised, his blood pressure is 180/85 mmHg, and his ECG shows sinus rhythm and voltage criteria for LVH.

What treatment would you consider to be least appropriate?

1. Start perindopril 2 mg
2. Low dose metoprolol
3. Start low dose nitrate
4. Commence a loop diuretic frusemide 20 mg
5. Do not start new medications and review in the OPD

A 63-year-old male who lives alone is referred with a short history of confusion and urinary incontinence. Eighteen months previously he had meningococcal meningitis that had responded well to penicillin. He is a lifelong non-smoker and drinks little alcohol. He lives alone but his daughter lives on the same street and cooks his meals.

On examination his temperature is 37°C, pulse 70/min regular, blood pressure 140/70 mmHg. He is alert and orientated in person but not in time or location. He is unable to remember simple sentences, and confabulates. His memory of recent events is poor. He is unable to perform simple arithmetic. There is no evidence of dysphasia, apraxia, or agnosia. There are no signs of meningism. Coordination in his lower limbs is poor; he has a wide-based, fixed-footed gait and tends to fall unless he has assistance. The remainder of the examination is unremarkable.

INVESTIGATIONS

Urinalysis	normal
Sodium	137 mmol/L
Potassium	3.7 mmol/L
Urea	7 mmol/L
Calcium	2.3 mmol/L
Albumin	38 g/L
Total protein	75 g/L
Urate	6.0 mmol/L
WBC	7×10^9/L
Platelets	400×10^9/L
ESR	30 mm in the first hour
Vitamin B_{12} and folate	normal
CRP	8 mg/L
VDRL	neg
T4	90 nmol/L
TSH	2.0 mU/L
Liver function tests including γ-GT	normal
Chest X-ray and skull X-ray	normal

a) What is the most likely diagnosis?
  1. Wernicke's encephalopathy
  2. Cerebellar infarct
  3. Normal pressure hydrocephalus
  4. Multiple sclerosis
  5. Alzeimer's disease

b) What is the treatment?
  1. Intravenous pabrinex and thiamine
  2. Aspirin
  3. Ventricular peritoneal shunt
  4. β interferon
  5. Surgery

Answer to Question 105 *is on page 320*

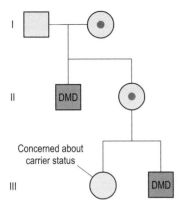

A 34-year-old female wishes to start a family with her partner. She has always believed she is a carrier for Duchenne muscular dystrophy (DMD) because a test performed as a teenager showed a raised creatine kinase level. She wants to know whether she carries the gene for DMD. Her uncle and brother were both affected (solid symbols) and her mother and grandmother are known to be carriers.

What is her chance of being a carrier?

1. 100%
2. 50%
3. 25%
4. Unable to ascertain
5. 75%

Answer to Question 106 *is on page 321*

A 16-year-old male presents with a history of recurrent chest infections since childhood. He has also suffered from recurrent sinus infections. On this occasion he has been increasingly short of breath for the last 3 days with a cough productive of copious purulent sputum.

a) Which of the following conditions would not be responsible for the clinical presentation?
  1. Kartagener's syndrome
  2. Hypogammaglobulinaemia
  3. Young's syndrome
  4. Cystic fibrosis
  5. C1-esterase inhibiter deficiency

b) The least likely organism to be isolated from the sputum would be:
  1. *Pseudomonas aeruginosa*
  2. *Haemophilus influenza*
  3. *Streptococcus milleri*
  4. *Staphylococcus aureus*
  5. *Aspergillus fumigatus*

A 44-year-old mother of three was referred from Greece for further treatment and investigation of possible systemic vasculitis. She presented 1 year previously with pain in her ankles and calves, which was particularly marked on exertion. She had a history of Raynaud's regular migraines and heavy menstrual periods. She drank 2 bottles of Retsina (Greek wine) per week. She was a life-long smoker of 20 cigarettes per day.

On examination the left radial pulse was absent, no pulses were felt below the femoral on the right, and the dorsalis pedis and posterior tibial were absent on the left. Blood pressure was normal and the peripheral perfusion was poor. She had localized ischaemia of the third toe on the right, with an interdigital infection.

INVESTIGATIONS

Hb 10.4 × 10^9/L, MCV 74 fL, ESR 23 mm/h, CRP 17 mg/L. Biochemical profile and blood glucose were normal. APTT and PT were normal. No antibodies to double stranded DNA were detectable; ANA was positive with a titre of 1/40; complement levels were normal. Anticardiolipin antibodies, lupus anticoagulant negative. Transthoracic ECHO was normal.

What is the likely diagnosis?

1. Antiphospholipid syndrome
2. Diabetes mellitus
3. Cholestrol emboli
4. Buerger's disease (thromboangitiis obliterans)
5. Cryoglobulinaemia

Answer to Question 108 *is on page 323*

A 45-year-old male is referred urgently by his GP with a clinical diagnosis of left lower lobe pneumonia, in association with a high fever and breathlessness. Previously the patient had undergone a renal transplant for Alport's syndrome at the age of 33 years. He is immunosuppressed with azathioprine. He had had two attacks of gout during the previous 6 weeks, and had been started on prophylactic treatment by the local rheumatologist.

Clinical examination confirms the GP's diagnosis, and a chest X-ray shows extensive left basal consolidation. Blood tests, performed urgently in A&E, reveal the following:

Hb	15 g/dL
WBC	0.7×10^9/L
Platelets	233×10^9/L
Sodium	136 mmol/L
Potassium	4 mmol/L
Urea	12 mmol/L
Creatinine	167 µmol/L
Bicarbonate	20 mmol/L
Calcium	2.4 mmol/L
Phosphate	1.0 mmol/L

What is the likely explanation for the full blood count results?

1. Leucopenia secondary to sepsis
2. Leucopenia secondary to allopurinol
3. Leucopenia secondary to azathioprine
4. Leucopenia secondary to colchicine
5. Leucopenia secondary to gout

A 28-year-old female has been found to have aortic stenosis. Her peak valve gradient is 70 mmHg. She wishes to start a family and has come to the clinic for advice.

On examination there are signs consistent with aortic stenosis. The left ventricle is not displaced and there are no other clinical signs of heart failure.

What would you advise her?

1. Antibiotic prophylaxis is needed but otherwise she may try for a family
2. She needs a metal valve replacement
3. She needs a tissue valve replacement
4. She should go forward for valvuloplasty
5. She should be commenced on an angiotensin converting enzyme inhibitor

Answer to Question 110 *is on page 325*

A 68-year-old male is admitted with acute severe chest pain. An ECG demonstrates changes consistent with myocardial infarction and he is thrombolyzed in the emergency department. His past history includes asthma; he infrequently takes a salbutamol inhaler. He is on no other medication.

On observation he is stable, pain free and his pulse is 78/min, blood pressure 138/70 mmHg and respiration rate 14/min.

His admission blood results show:

Hb	13.2 g/dL
WCC	6.8×10^9/L
Platelets	340×10^9/L
Sodium	134 mmol/L
Potassium	4.2 mmol/L
Urea	7.8 mmol/L
Creatinine	120 mmol/L
Glucose	11.1 mmol/L

What would be your next management step?

1. Commence beta blocker – atenolol 25 mg
2. Institute insulin – dextrose sliding scale
3. Commence a statin
4. Start a glycoprotein IIa/IIIb inhibitor
5. Start gliclazide 40 mg bd

A 35-year-old female patient is being investigated for hypertension. All her medication had been stopped. This is her ECG:

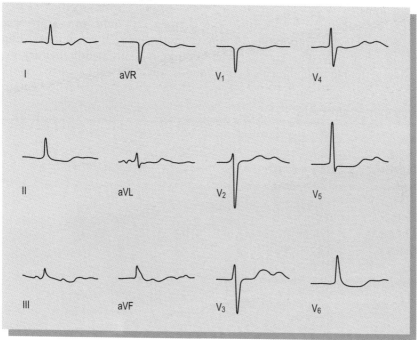

What underlying diagnosis would you consider?

1. Acromegaly
2. Coarctation of the aorta
3. Fibromuscular dysplasia of the renal arteries
4. Conn's syndrome
5. Essential hypertension with left ventricular hypertrophy

A 40-year-old male is admitted with a suspected overdose. He is unresponsive and has been intubated. A bottle of amitriptyline tablets was found beside him.

On examination: temperature 36.5°C, pulse 100/min, blood pressure 120/80 mmHg, respiration rate 14/min (ventilated); pupils 4 mm fixed, deep tendon reflexes ++, plantars ⇓⇓. Other findings: mucous membranes dry ++, bladder palpable to umbilicus, bowel sounds soft.

INVESTIGATIONS

Hb	14.2 g/dL
WCC	12.1 × 10⁹/L
Platelets	286 × 10⁹/L
Sodium	130 mmol/L
Potassium	4.8 mmol/L
Urea	9.8 mmol/L
Creatinine	99 µmol/L
Glucose	4.8 mmol/L
Cl	91 mmol/L

Blood gases on ventilation

pH	7.3
pCO_2	3.1 kPa
PO_2	20 kPa
Bicarbonate	9 mmol/L
	Urine crystalluria

What are these results consistent with?

1. Amitriptyline overdose only
2. Combined amitriptyline and ethanol overdose
3. Combined amitriptyline and ethylene glycol overdose
4. Amitriptyline and opiate overdose
5. Amitriptyline and benzodiazepine overdose

Answer to Question 113 *is on page 328*

A 56-year-old train driver presents with a 2-week history of diffuse arthralgia, fatigue and a dry non-productive cough. He saw his GP 3 days previously who prescribed a course of antibiotics but his symptoms have worsened.

On examination his temperature is 37.5°C, pulse 100/min, respiration rate 22/min, blood pressure 110/60 mmHg. A 1.5-cm lymph node is palpable in his neck. His respiratory examination is normal. Abdominal examination reveals hepatosplenomegaly. On examination of his gums you notice that they are hypertrophied.

What is the most likely diagnosis?

1. Lymphoma
2. Mycoplasma pneumonia
3. Acute myelomonocytic leukaemia (M4).
4. Tuberculosis
5. Acute lymphoblastic leukaemia

A 35-year-old male solicitor is referred by his GP. He had been diagnosed as being hypertensive 1 year previously and despite drug treatment including beta blockers, calcium antagonists and an ACE inhibitor, his blood pressure remains elevated. His general health is excellent; he drinks 4 pints of beer per day and smokes 2 cigars every evening.

In the clinic, supine blood pressure is recorded as 210/110 mmHg. Fundi – grade III hypertensive retinopathy. The rest of the examination is normal.

INVESTIGATIONS

Sodium	148 mmol/L
Potassium	3.0 mmol/L
Bicarbonate	32 mmol/L
Urea	4 mmol/IL
Creatinine	109 umol/L
Glucose	4 mmol/L
Urine	negative protein and blood

a) What is the likely diagnosis?
1. poor compliance
2. ectopic ACTH production
3. Primary hyperaldosteronism (Conn's syndrome)
4. phaeochromocytoma
5. hypernephroma

b) Which further investigation is required to make an endocrinological diagnosis?
1. USS kidneys
2. MRA of kidneys
3. 24-h urinary cateocholamines
4. Serum aldosterone and renin (supine samples)
5. Venous sampling of adrenal glands
6. MIBG scan
7. CT scan of adrenals

Question 116

A 56-year-old male treated for mycobacterial tuberculosis for 9 months complains of numb feet. Nerve conduction studies show the following:

Sural sensory action potential	8 µV (normal >15 µV)
Median nerve sensory action potential	4 µV (normal > 20 µV)
Common peroneal motor nerve velocity	48 m/s (normal >45 m/s)

a) What type of neuropathy is present?
   1. A demyelinating neuropathy
   2. A motor neuropathy
   3. A sensory neuropathy
   4. Axonal neuropathy
   5. Mixed axonal demyelinating pattern

b) What is the likely explanation in this patient?
   1. Pyrazinamide induced
   2. Rifampicin induced
   3. Isoniazid induced
   4. Ethambutol induced
   5. Streptomycin induced

Answer to Question 116 *is on page 332*

A 50-year-old unemployed insurance clerk is admitted for further assessment. He is known to be a heavy alcohol drinker.

The positive features on examination are that he is jaundiced, he has hepatomegaly, evidence of ascites and he has pitting oedema to his sacrum.

Sodium	118 mmol/L
Potassium	4.6 mmol/L
Urea	10.0 mmol/L
Creatinine	84 µmol/L
Bilirubin	166 µmol/L
ALP	175 iu/L
AST	371 iu/L
Albumin	24 g/L
Total protein	72 g/L
Globulin	48 g/L
INR	2.0
Glucose	5.8 mmol/L
CRP	10 mg/L
Bicarbonate	20 mmol/L
Hb	12.2 g/dL
WCC	5.8×10^9/L
Platelets	320×10^9/L

As part of his inpatient assessment he has an endoscopy which reveals Grade II oesophageal varices.

a) The initial treatment should be:
1. Oral propanolol
2. Variceal band ligation
3. No treatment and re-endoscope in 1 year
4. Variceal sclerotherapy
5. Liver transplantation

b) What is the likely cause of the hyponatraemia in this patient?
1. Polydipsia
2. Syndrome of inappropriate antidiuretic hormone
3. Secondary to cirrhosis
4. Secondary to diuretics
5. Addison's disease

Answer to Question 117 *is on page 333*

Question 118

A 57-year-old male has been given a diagnosis of amyotrophic lateral sclerosis.

a) Which two of the following would be least compatible with this diagnosis?
   1. The presence of any abnormality on MR imaging
   2. A creatinine kinase level of 1500 iu
   3. Involvement of eye movements
   4. Sensory changes on nerve conduction studies
   5. No evidence of upper motor neuron involvement
   6. Normal lumber puncture results
   7. Normal nerve conduction velocity

b) For which of the following is there an evidence base that it may prolong life?
   1. Riluzole
   2. High dose vitamin E
   3. Physiotherapy
   4. B-interferon
   5. Glial-derived neurotrophic factor

Answer to Question 118 *is on page 334*

A 30-year-old female presents with palpitations and chest pain. On auscultation there is a midsystolic click and a late systolic murmur.

Which of the following statements is correct?

1. An echocardiogram may show abrupt displacement of both mitral valve leaflets
2. Her ECG is likely to show lateral ischaemic changes
3. The click and murmur should occur later in systole when she stands up
4. Spontaneous bacterial endocarditis is rare and prophylactic antibiotics are not recommended
5. She is likely to have an underlying connective tissue disorder

Answer to Question 119 *is on page 335*

A 20-year-old female presents to the outpatient department with widespread bruising and bleeding gums.

Blood results are as follows:

Hb	9.2 g/dL	
WCC	20.4 × 10⁹/L	80% myeloblasts, 8% promyelocytes, 7% neutrophils
Platelets	20 × 10⁹/L	
PT	23 s	
APPT	70 s	
Fibrinogen	0.78 g/L	
TT	20 s	15–19 s

a) What is the likely underlying diagnosis?
   1. Acute promyelocytic leukaemia
   2. Lymphoma
   3. Acute lymphoblastic leukemia
   4. Idiopathic thrombocytopenic purpura
   5. Septicaemia

b) The most important investigation would be:
   1. Vitamin B_{12}, folate and iron
   2. Bone marrow examination
   3. Philadelphia chromosome
   4. Coombs' test
   5. CT scan of chest abdomen and pelvis

Answer to Question 120 *is on page 336*

A 76-year-old male has a 3-month history of weight loss, anorexia and fever. He has also been complaining of increased urinary frequency. He has been a lifelong smoker of 10-20 cigarettes per day and has always had an early morning cough productive of grey phlegm.

Examination is unremarkable aside from some swelling of the lower limbs.

INVESTIGATIONS

Hb	18.2 g/dL
WCC	10 × 10⁹/L
Platelets	300 × 10⁹/L
Sodium	140 mmol/L
Potassium	3.1 mmol/L
Urea	7.0 mmol/L
Creatinine	115 µmol/L
Calcium	2.9 mmol/L
Urinalysis	Blood +++

What is the most likely diagnosis?

1. Squamous cell carcinoma of the lung
2. Oat cell carcinoma of the lung
3. Lymphoma
4. Renal cell carcinoma
5. Renal tuberculosis

A 32-year-old male is admitted with palpitations that have occurred since the previous evening. He has never had an episode prior to this. He has no family history of heart disease. He does not smoke or drink alcohol. On examination he is anxious but not breathless. His blood pressure is 155/74 mmHg.

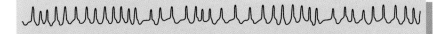

a) From the following what is the most likely diagnosis?
   1. Atrial flutter with 2:1 block
   2. Atrial fibrillation with pre-excitation
   3. Torsades de pointes
   4. Polymorphic ventricular tachycardia
   5. Orthodromic atrioventricular re-entrant tachycardia

b) Which treatment would you use?
   1. IV verapamil
   2. IV adenosine
   3. IV atropine
   4. IV flecainide
   5. DC cardioversion

Answer to Question 122 *is on page 339*

A 24-year-old male presents with bluish discolouration of the body, lips and nails, which has been evident from birth. General examination reveals the presence of central cyanosis with steel grey complexion of the body. He is not clubbed. Cardiorespiratory examination is otherwise normal.

Investigations show a haemoglobin of 17 g/dL and normal blood biochemistry. The arterial blood gas analysis reveals a PaO2 of 110 mmHg and an oxygen saturation of 90%.

What is the diagnosis?

1. Methaemoglobinaemia
2. Haemochromatosis
3. Congenital cyanotic heart disease
4. Stress polycythaemia
5. Polcythaemia rubra vera

Answer to Question 123 *is on page 340*

Question 124

A 20-year-old female undergoes assessment for increasing dyspnoea. Examination is unremarkable apart from a soft systolic murmur at the left sternal edge and a widely split second heart sound.

Her electrocardiogram, cardiac catheterization and oxygen saturations are shown below.

Cardiac catheterization data:

Anatomical site	Oxygen saturation
SVC	76%
IVC	74%
RA(high)	73%
RA(mid)	80%
RA(low)	81%
RV	82%
PA	81%
LV	96%
Aorta	96%

Electrocardiogram:

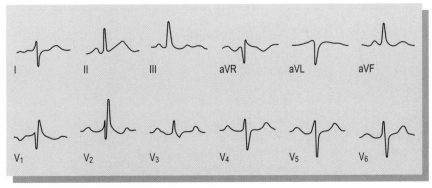

a) What two abnormalities are apparent on this ECG?
   1. Atrial fibrillation
   2. Lateral T-wave inversion
   3. Left axis deviation
   4. Left bundle branch block
   5. Right axis deviation
   6. Right bundle branch block
   7. Sinus arrest
   8. ST segment depression

b) What is likely to be the diagnosis?
   1. Mitral valve prolapse
   2. Osteum primum atrial septal defect
   3. Osteum secundum atrial septal defect
   4. Aortic stenosis
   5. Ventricular septal defect

Answer to Question 124 *is on page 341*

A 72-year-old male is admitted complaining of severe polyarticular joint pain. During the previous week the GP has had to visit on a number of occasions because of a possible lower respiratory tract infection. The patient has had osteoarthritis of the knees for 10 years and has been diagnosed with myelodysplasia.

2 months prior to admission his GP had stopped his non-steriodal anti-inflammatory drugs (NSAIDs) because of a possible coffee ground vomit. He lives alone, drinks about 25 units of alcohol per week and has been a lifelong smoker. Current medications: ferrous sulphate 200 mg tds, quinine sulphate 300 mg nocte.

On examination: pulse 100/min, respiratory rate 13/min, blood pressure 150/90 mmHg, temperature 36.4°C. Both wrists, both knees, both ankles, the 2nd and 3rd metacarpophalangeal joints of the right hand, and the 3rd and 5th distal phalangeal joints of the left hand, are red, swollen and painful. Respiratory examination demonstrates some coarse crepitations at the left base. Respiratory and cardiovascular examination was normal.

INVESTIGATIONS

Hb	9.4 g/dL
WCC	13.2 (neut 6) $\times 10^9$/L
Platelets	100 $\times 10^9$/L
CRP	280 Mg/L
Sodium	130 mmol/L
Potassium	4.8 mmol/L
Urea	36 mmol/L
Creatinine*	240 µmol/L
Rheumatoid factor	strongly positive
ANA	weakly positive

*Note: previous results indicate a consistent renal dysfunction

Aspiration of the knee: no organisms, negatively birifrigent crystals under polarized light.

a) What is the likely cause of the joint pains?
1. Rheumatoid arthritis
2. Pseudogout
3. Gout
4. Mycoplasma pneumonia
5. Reactive arthritis

Question continued overpage

He was rehydrated, but still had severe joint pain despite the use of opiates and colchicine 500 mcg bd.

b) What treatment would you consider most appropriate?
1. Start oral prednisolone
2. Start allopurinol
3. Increase the dose of colchicine to 500 mcg 4-hourly
4. Commence a COX II inhibitor
5. Commence antibiotics

Answer to Question 125 *is on page 342*

A 54-year-old male has been thrombolyzed with streptokinase for an acute myocardial infarction. Forty minutes after thrombolysis he is still in pain. He is fully conscious, there are no clinical signs of cardiac failure and his blood pressure is 98/60 mmHg.

According to the best evidence-based practice, what treatment should he have?

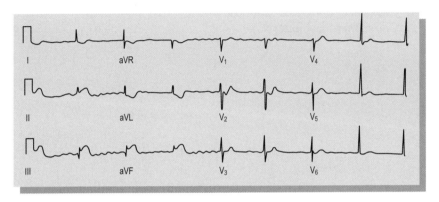

1. Immediate re-thrombolysis with streptokinase
2. Immediate re-thrombolysis with a recombinant tissue plasminogen activator
3. Rescue angioplasty
4. Continue current regimen and monitor closely
5. Urgent cardiac surgery

Answer to Question 126 *is on page 343*

A 60-year-old female presents to the acute medical team with a history of sudden shortness of breath. She had been admitted 12 months previously with an inferior myocardial infarction, and since then she has been admitted on at least five occasions with similar symptoms. On each occasion she was treated medically with a combination of diuretics, nitrates and oxygen from which she usually made a good recovery. Review of the notes shows that she has had a previous femoral-popliteal bypass. An echocardiogram shows mild impairment of left ventricular contraction and aortic stenosis (valve gradient 25 mm/Lg). In between admissions she remained well, but her GP had again referred her to the cardiology clinic for control of her blood pressure.

INVESTIGATIONS

Hb	13.8 mmol/L
WCC	10.3 × 10^9/L
Platelets	184 × 10^9/L
Sodium	137 mmol/L
Potassium	3.6 mmol/L
Urea	11.1 mmol/L
Creatinine	218 μmol/L
Glucose	4.8 mmol/L
Albumin	38 g/L
Chol	8.6 mmol/L
Tryglceride	2.2 mmol/L
Urinalysis	no protein/blood

a) What is the most likely underlying diagnosis?
   1. Constrictive pericarditis
   2. Aortic stenosis
   3. Brittle asthma
   4. Atherosclerotic renal artery stenosis
   5. Recurrent pulmonary emboli

b) How would you investigate her further in the first instance?
   1. Renal ultrasound
   2. V/Q scan
   3. D-dimers
   4. Cardiac catheterization
   5. Formal lung function tests and sequential a.m. and p.m. peak flow recordings

Answer to Question 127 *is on page 344*

A 65-year-old female develops persistent diarrhoea. On examination she appears to have a migratory erythematous rash over her legs.

INVESTIGATIONS

Hb	9 g/dL
WBC	11×10^9/L
Platelets	230×10^9/L
Fasting glucose	10 mmol/L

a) Give a unifying diagnosis:
1. Thyrotoxicosus
2. Cushing's disease
3. Conn's syndrome
4. Glucagonoma
5. Chronic pancreatitis

b) How would you confirm your diagnosis?
1. Elevated serum amylase
2. Raised fasting glucagon levels
3. Thyroid function tests
4. Abdominal CT scan
5. 24 hour urine free cortisol measurement

A 55-year-old male presents with fatigue, lethargy, loss of weight and night sweats. His admission was precipitated by sudden left-sided abdominal and shoulder tip pain. Examination reveals exquisite tenderness over that area and a palpable spleen 10 cm below the costal margin. There is no lymphadenopathy or jaundice.

Blood results are as follows:

Hb	6.3 g/dL	
WCC	53×10^9/L	
Platelets	530×10^9/L	
Neut	56%	
Lymphocytes	1%	
Monocytes	1%	
Eosinophils	3%	
Basophils	3%	
NAP score	24	NR (35–100)

What is the most likely diagnosis?

1. Myelodysplasia
2. Acute myeloid leukaemia
3. Multiple myeloma
4. Leukaemoid reaction
5. Chronic myeloid leukaemia

Answer to Question 129 *is on page 346*

A 64-year-old Somali female has a 6-month history of a weight loss of 2 stones, and episodic severe colicky abdominal pain that is not associated with meals, posture or bowel habit.

INVESTIGATIONS

Sodium	125 mmol/L
Potassium	6.4 mmol/L
Urea	14 mmol/l
Calcium	2.76 mmol/L
Glucose	3.3 mmol/L
T4	8 nmol/L
TSH	10 mU/L
Thyroid microsomal antibodies	not detected

a) What is the most likely diagnosis?
   1. Hypopituitarism
   2. Multiple endocrine neoplasia type I
   3. Autoimmune adrenal failure
   4. Primary hypothyroidism
   5. Adrenal failure secondary to tuberculosis

b) What treatment is indicated for the endocrine abnormalities?
   1. Hydrocortisone and fludrocortisone
   2. Carbimazole
   3. Thyroxine
   4. Prednisolone
   5. Glucagon

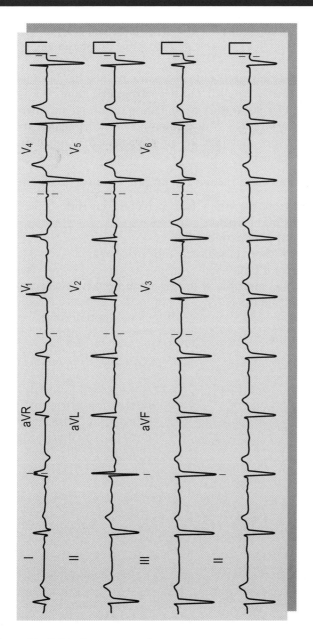

What does this ECG demonstrate?

1. Left anterior hemi block
2. Right axis deviation
3. Old inferior myocardial infarction
4. Bifascicular block
5. Trifascicular block

An 80-year-old female has suffered a dense left-sided cerebrovascular event. This has resulted in an expressive and receptive dysphasia and a right-sided hemiparesis.

Swallowing was impaired and nasogastric feeding has been initiated. On three occasions she has pulled out her nasogastric tube. She is otherwise alert and stable. Her respiratory examination is normal and there is no current evidence of aspiration. A discussion between the healthcare team and her family establishes that they are in agreement that nutritional support should currently continue.

Which of the following is the most appropriate course of action?

1. Seek consent from the family for a percutaneous endoscopic gastrostomy (PEG) insertion
2. Start peripheral parenteral feeding
3. Arrange for fine bore nasogastric tube placement
4. Sign consent for a PEG
5. Arrange for PEG insertion with consent in her best interests, by her nominated consultant

Answer to Question 132 *is on page 351*

Question 133

A 27-year-old female American tourist is admitted with rapidly progressive weakness. This initially started with pain in the arms and legs, which was followed by a tingling sensation in the feet, and which rapidly spread to involve the legs, arms and face. Two weeks previously, before leaving Colorado, she had had an episode of diarrhoea and abdominal pain, which took several days to settle.

On examination she was apyrexial and had: a pulse of 90/min regular, blood pressure 150/80 mmHg lying and 120/60 mmHg sitting, respiratory rate 22/min. The chest was clear, cranial nerve examination was normal, she had a flaccid weakness of the legs and arms (MRC grade 3/5), her reflexes were not present, and her plantars were flexor.

INVESTIGATIONS

CSF	Finding
Appearance	clear, colourless
Leukocytes	1
Microorganisms	none
Culture	negative
Glucose (mmol/L)	2.8
Protein (g/L)	2.6
Blood	
FBC, urea and electrolytes	normal
glucose	3.8 mmol/L

a) What is the most likely diagnosis?
1. Neurological presentation of Lyme disease
2. Guillain–Barré syndrome (acute inflammatory demyelinating polyneuropathy)
3. Myasthenia gravis
4. Botulism
5. Multiple sclerosis

The day after admission she continued to deteriorate: her swallowing was judged to be unsafe, she had facial weakness and she had increasing difficulty breathing. Her forced vital capacity was measured at 1.2 Litres.

b) What two other treatment options would you institute at this stage?
1. IV immunoglobulin
2. Sedation and intubation
3. IV methylprednisolone
4. Plasma exchange
5. Broad spectrum antibiotics
6. Non-invasive positive pressure ventilation
7. Close observation and supportive treatment

Answer to Question 133 *is on page 352*

A 65-year-old female presents with a 2-year history of arthralgia and a raised purpuric rash affecting her legs over the last 2 months. She has also suffered from severe pain in her hands particularly when they are exposed to the cold. There was no other relevant history.

INVESTIGATIONS

Hb	13.2 g/dL
WCC	6.8×10^9/L
Platelets	140×10^9/L
Sodium	138 mmol/L
Potassium	4.3 mmol/L
Urea	6.1 mmol/L
Creatinine	140 µmol/L
Glucose	5.1 mmol/L
CRP	4 µg/L

RF positive, ANA weak positive
Complement: normal C3 and low C4
24-h protein: 3.1 g /24 h

What is the most likely underlying diagnosis?

1. SLE
2. Cryoglobulinaemia
3. Polyarteritis nodosa
4. Raynaud's disease
5. Wegener's granulomatosis

Answer to Question 134 *is on page 354*

A 68-year-old female had been admitted to the CCU with an anterior myocardial infarction 24 hours previously. She was making a good recovery but suddenly her condition deteriorated and she became acutely short of breath with severe chest pain.

On examination she is clammy and shut down and has a blood pressure reading of 90/70 mmHg. There is a previously undetected harsh systolic murmur heard loudest over the left sternal edge with an accentuated second sound. The lung fields are clear.

a) What is the most likely diagnosis?
  1. Rupture of the ventricular free wall
  2. Papillary muscle rupture
  3. Ventricular septal rupture
  4. Pericardial tamponade
  5. Dressler's syndrome

b) What would be the most appropriate intervention?
  1. Cardiac angiography
  2. Immediate consideration for surgery
  3. Re-thrombolysis
  4. Supportive management
  5. Initial conservative management and surgical consideration in 1–3 weeks

A 34-year-old mother with a diagnosis of Osteogenesis imperfecta brings her 12-year-old son into the clinic. He wants to play rugby at school and she is concerned that he too may have Osteogenesis imperfecta. To date he has had no injuries and is tall for his age. Her 6-year-old daughter has had multiple fractures throughout childhood. The mother, however, is an orphan and no other family history is available.

What would you advise her?

1. Tell her that the condition is X-linked recessive and that he would have died in early childhood if he was affected
2. Screen initially with bone mineral densitrometry T scores
3. Request genetic linkage analysis
4. Screen with urinary calcium excretion
5. Request serum calcium, phosphate and alkaline phosphatase
6. Send dermal punch biopsies for collagen biochemical analysis

Answer to Question 136 *is on page 358*

A 72-year-old male presents with sudden onset of weakness in his right leg and arm and bumping into things on that side. His past history includes a short-lived period of aphasia 7 months previously from which he made a full recovery. Medications: bendrofluazide 2.5 mg.

On examination he is alert and orientated, with a pulse of 78/min regular and blood pressure 160/85 mmHg. General systems examination is normal and there is no carotid bruit. On central nervous system examination he has a right homonymous visual field defect and reduced power in the right upper and lower limbs.

An emergency CT head scan shows no abnormality. An ECG shows SR borderline 1st degree heart block.

a) What vascular territory is likely to have been involved?
   1. Middle and anterior cerebral artery territory
   2. Vertebrobasilar circulation
   3. Anterior cerebral artery territory
   4. Posterior inferior cerebellar artery
   5. Lacunar territory

b) Which of the following investigations would you perform next?
   1. Echocardiogram
   2. Carotid Doppler of neck vessels
   3. MRI angiogram of the brain
   4. CT chest
   5. 24-h tape

Answer to Question 137 *is on page 359*

A 54-year-old bricklayer has had increasing difficulty climbing his ladder at work and has noted increasing joint stiffness in the morning. He has a past history of pancreatitis, a right calf deep vein thrombosis following a fractured tibia, hypothyroidism and psoriasis. Current medication is thyroxine 125 mcg od. His social history: admits to illicit anabolic steroid use, alcohol – 60 units/week. He has smoked 20 cigarettes per day for 20 years.

On examination he has global muscle tenderness with an erythematous rash affecting the periorbital regions and dorsum of the hands.

a) From the following, which three would be the most useful in establishing a diagnosis?
1. EMG
2. Serum creatinine kinase
3. Urine screen for anabolic steroids
4. 24-h urinary cortisol excretion
5. CRP
6. Serum anti-Sm antibody
7. MRI scan of the right thigh
8. urine and faecal porphyrin estimations
9. Immunoglobulins + protein strip

b) What is the likely diagnosis?
1. Dermatomyositis
2. McArdle's disease
3. Psoriatic arthropathy
4. Polmyalgia rheumatica
5. Myopathy secondary to anabolic steroids
6. Mycosis fungoides
7. Porphyria cutanea tarda

A 60-year-old female is admitted to hospital with a history of palpitations during the 90 min prior to admission. Over the previous year this had occurred on three occasions and during the episodes she felt unwell but had not lost consciousness.

She is comfortable while the following trace is taken.

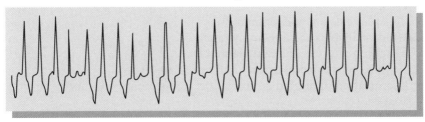

Her heart rate is 160/min with a blood pressure of 120/70 mmHg.

What is the diagnosis?

1. Ventricular fibrillation
2. Atrial fibrillation
3. Supraventricular tachycardia with abherrent conduction
4. Wolff-Parkinson-White
5. Ventricular tachycardia

A 58-year-old female patient has been diagnosed with polymyalgia rheumatica and has been started on prednisolone 15 mg daily. She has had a good response to treatment over the last couple of months.

Which one of the following options would you initiate to prevent steroid-induced osteoporosis?

1. HRT plus calcium and vitamin D
2. Alendronate plus calcium and vitamin D
3. Calcitonin plus calcium and vitamin D
4. Measure bone mineral density and review in 1 year
5. Treatment not indicated at present because steroids will shortly be stopped

A 50-year-old female is admitted with recent onset of dysphagia for liquids with nasal regurgitation. Her friends have commented that she has an expressionless face.

Which test could you perform at the bedside to elucidate a cause?

1. Elicit a jaw jerk
2. Look at the tongue for fasciculation
3. Count numbers out aloud
4. Shake the patient's hand
5. Test the reflexes

A 17-year-old male is referred from his GP with a purpuric rash on his legs. The clinic sister has just dipped his urine and it reveals proteinuria + and haematuria +++.

What is the most likely diagnosis?

1. Henoch-Schönlein purpura
2. Mixed essential cryoglobulinaemia
3. Minimal change nephropathy
4. IgA nephropathy
5. Membranous glomerulonephritis

A 72-year-old male residing in England but having moved from Bangladesh 5 years previously presents with a 3-month history of abdominal distension, malaise and anorexia. His past history includes type II diabetes and ulcerative colitis. Current medication is glicazide and aspirin.

Examination reveals abdominal signs consistent with moderate ascites and a palpable liver edge 3 cm below the costal margin. There are no other peripheral stigmata of liver disease and the patient is not jaundiced. Blood pressure is 120/70 mmHg, respiratory rate 14/min, pulse 80/min regular, O_2 saturation 98% air.

Blood results are as follows:

Sodium	141 mmol/L	γ-GT	307 iu/L
Urea	6.1 mmol/L	Glucose	11.6 mmol/L
Creatinine	91 μmol/L		
Calcium	2.3 mmol/L	Hb	13.4 g/dL
Albumin	34 g/L	WCC	9.8×10^9/L
Bilirubin	21 μmol/L	Platelets	141×10^9/L
ALP	141 iu/L	INR	1.3
AST	59 iu/L	APTT	17.1s

Hepatitis serology: anti-hep C Ab (+)

a) Which three other tests would you request at this stage:
 1. Alpha-feto protein levels
 2. CT abdomen
 3. Hepatic ultrasound and Doppler studies
 4. Mantoux test
 5. Alpha-1-antitrypsin levels
 6. Liver biopsy
 7. Hepatitis C PCR

b) Which one of the following would you select to manage his ascites?
 1. Start a loop diuretic and spironolactone
 2. Therapeutic paracentesis albumin replacement
 3. Advise salt and fluid restriction
 4. Recommend bed rest and continue with investigations
 5. Start spironolactone

Answer to Question 143 *is on page 366*

A 59-year-old divorced social worker is referred from his GP with a long history of low back pain and increased urinary frequency. The GP was also concerned that the patient had visited her on a number of occasions seeking early retirement because his colleagues found him sometimes vague at work. He is not on regular medications. He smokes 20 cigarettes and drinks two pints of beer per day.

Examination is unremarkable apart from some minimal tenderness over the lumbosacral spine. Plain X-ray imaging has been reported as normal.

The GP is concerned about the following results:

Hb	13.2 g/dL	ALP	48 iu/L
MCV	85 fL	ALT	50 iu/L
WBC	8.2×10^9/L	Albumin	34 g/L
Platelets	287×10^9/L		
ESR	20 mm in first hour	IgG	18 g/L (IgG monoclonal band)
Sodium	134 mmol/L	IgM	0.8 g/L
Potassium	3.9 mmol/L	IgA	2.5 g/L
Urea	8.0 mmol/L		
Creatinine	99 µmol/L	Bence-Jones protein	negative
Glucose	4.5 mmol/L		
Calcium (corrected)	2.3 mmol/L	Skeletal survey	normal
Bicarbonate	20 mmol/L		
Cl	90 mmol/L		

How would you account for the above thus far?

1. Reactive depression
2. Benign paraproteinaemia
3. Myelofibrosis
4. Myeloma
5. Waldenström's macroglobinaemia

A 35-year-old female presents with swollen ankles. Subsequent investigation shows her to have a 24-h urine protein level of 7 g in 24 h.

What is the most probable renal diagnosis?

1. Focal segmental glomerulosclerosis
2. Minimal change disease
3. Membranous glomerulosclerosis
4. IgA nephropathy
5. Mesangiocapillary glomerulonephritis

Answer to Question 145 *is on page 370*

An 18-year-old male who has previously been fit and is on no medication becomes unwell with fever, myalgia, loss of appetite and a sore throat. His GP diagnoses viral tonsilitis. On review 48 h later he is concerned that the patient is clinically jaundiced and refers him to casualty.

INVESTIGATIONS:

Hb	14.8 g/dL
MCV	88 fL
Reticulocytes	1%
WBC	6×10^9/L
Platelets	259×10^9/L
ESR	10 mm in the first hour
Bilirubin	55 µmol/L
Conjugated bilirubin	9 µmol/L
Aspartate aminotransferase	25 iu/L
Alkaline phosphatase	105 iu/L
Albumin	42 g/L
Urea and electrolytes	normal

What is the likely diagnosis?

1. Crigler–Najjar syndrome
2. Dubin–Johnson syndrome
3. Gilbert's syndrome
4. Rotor syndrome
5. Haemolytic anaemia

Answer to Question 146 *is on page 371*

A 77-year-old retired army colonel is referred by his GP with a history of increasing limb stiffness and a mild resting tremor; he has also noticed that his writing has become very small and unreadable. These symptoms have progressed over the preceding 3 to 4 years. Over the previous year he has also developed hallucinations and confusion; he wakes up at night shouting at people apparently invading the garden. He often gets lost in the house and has taken to hiding food in the library. He is on no regular medication, has been a lifelong non-smoker and does not drink alcohol.

On examination he is confused in time and place. His blood pressure is 130/100 mmHg and there is no postural drop. He has symmetrical rigidity with a mild tremor in both the arms and legs. Cranial nerve examination shows mild restriction of conjugate up gaze. He has a festinant gait, which is unstable with a tendency to fall backwards.

What is the most likely diagnosis?

1. Progressive supranuclear palsy
2. Olivopontocerebellar degeneration
3. Lewy body dementia
4. Post-traumatic stress disorder
5. Idiopathic Parkinson's disease
6. Vascular dementia

Answer to Question 147 *is on page 373*

A 53-year-old Maltese female is being investigated for a 4-year history of intermittant puffiness around the eyes, a flitting arthralgia, Raynaud's phenomenon, a right median nerve palsy and, more recently, she has had intermittent diarrhoea and abdominal pain precipitating her admission. She has had no prior illnesses, does not drink or smoke and has no positive family history. Examination reveals her to be normotensive, and confirms the presence of a petechial vasculitic rash on her trunk and flexor surfaces. She has weakness and wasting in the median nerve distribution in the right hand. The clinic sister has performed a urine dipstick and it is negative.

What is the most likely diagnosis?

1. Wegener's granulomatosis
2. Kawasaki disease
3. Henoch-Schönlein purpura
4. C1-esterase deficiency
5. Polyarteritis nodosa

Answer to Question 148 *is on page 375*

A 32-year-old salesman presents to a follow-up clinic with an 8-week history of night sweats sufficient to soak the sheets, and right upper quadrant pain. He has lost 6 kg in 3 months and is drinking 2 pints of beer daily. On examination he is pyrexial, with a temperature of 38.3°C, thin and pale with four-fingers' breadth of tender hepatomegaly. He has no lymphadenopathy and is not icteric.

Past medical history: Hodgkin's disease stage III diagnosed 1 year previously, treated with combined chemotherapy.

INVESTIGATIONS

Hb	11.8 g/dL
WBC	2.4×10^9/L – 70% neutrophils
Platelets	345×10^9/L
Sodium	139 mmol/L
Potassium	4.5 mmol/L
Bicarbonate	27 mmol/L
Creatinine	87 µmol/L
Alkaline phosphatase	372 iu/L
Aspartate transaminase	79 iu/L
Bilirubin	24 µmol/L
Albumin	36 g/L
Protein	72 g/L
Chest X-ray	diffuse bilateral infiltration with occasional nodules

a) What is the most likely diagnosis now?
1. Myelofibrosis and secondary sepsis
2. Tuberculosis
3. Hepatic abscess
4. Recurrent lymphoma with *Pneumocystis carinii* pneumonia
5. Sarcoidosis

b) Choose three diagnostic procedures:
1. Heaf test
2. Bronchoscopy with washings and transbronchial biopsy
3. Bone marrow
4. CT scan of abdomen
5. Liver biopsy
6. Gallium scan
7. Lymph node biopsy

A 59-year-old female presents to the outpatient department with increasing tiredness, nausea and thirst. She has frequent epigastric pain and has woken on three occasions in the night with such pain in the previous week.

INVESTIGATIONS

Hb	11.8 g/dL
WBC	6.4×10^9/L
Platelets	264×10^9/L
ESR	9 mm in the first hour
Sodium	136 mmol/L
Potassium	4.3 mmol/L
Urea	11.5 mmol/L
Creatinine	140 µmol/L
Calcium	3.25 mmol/L
Phosphate	0.72 mmol/L (0.8–1.4)
Chloride	117 mmol/L (90–110)
Bicarbonate	12 mmol/L (20–30)
Alkaline phosphatase	170 iu/L
Albumin	40 g/L
Total protein	80 g/L (60–80)

a) What is the likely diagnosis?
   1. Multiple myeloma
   2. Bony metatases
   3. Primary hyperparathyroidism
   4. Tertiary hyperparathyroidism
   5. Chronic renal failure

b) What is the significance of the epigastric pain?
   1. Acute pancreatitis
   2. Liver secondaries
   3. Peptic ulceration
   4. Myocardial ischaemia
   5. Pulmonary embolism

c) How would you confirm your diagnosis?
   1. Serum electrophoresis
   2. Bone marrow examination
   3. Bone scan
   4. Skeletal survey
   5. Measure parathyroid hormone levels

Answer to Question 150 *is on page 378*

A 40-year-old Chinese male, who is otherwise fit and well, is admitted for a hernia repair. He has lived and worked in the UK for 25 years. He drinks no alcohol and takes no herbal remedies or other medications. He has no history of illness in the past and has never had a blood transfusion. The following blood results are obtained:

Sodium	140 mmol/L
Potassium	4.0 mmol/L
Urea	6 mmol/L
Albumin	40 mg/L
AST	120 iu/L
ALP	140 iu/L
Bilirubin	10 µmol/L
HBs Ag	positive
HBe Ag	positive
HBcIgG Ab	positive
ANA	negative

a) What is the likely diagnosis?
   1. Acute hepatitis B infection
   2. Chronic active hepatitis
   3. Acute hepatitis E infection
   4. Chronic hepatitis B infection with low infectivity
   5. Chronic hepatitis B infection with high infectivity

b) What are the indications for treatment? Name two:
   1. Cirrhosis on liver biopsy
   2. Development of HBe Ab
   3. Chronic active hepatitis on liver biopsy
   4. Cirrhosis on liver ultrasound
   5. HBV DNA polymerase detected in the serum

Answer to Question 151 *is on page 380*

A 38-year-old female presents with a haematoma over her left elbow and an INR of 14 measured at the GP surgery. She takes warfarin for a previous pulmonary embolus and three deep vein thromboses. There is no family history of a clotting disorder and she has had two uneventful pregnancies.

Examination confirms the haematoma and no other source of bleeding; her observations are stable. The remainder of her blood results are normal.

What would your treatment be?

1. Fresh frozen plasma 2 units
2. No treatment
3. Platelet transfusion
4. Vitamin K 1 mg IV
5. Give prothrombin concentrate

Answer to Question 152 *is on page 381*

A 30-year-old doctor presents for urgent review in the diabetic clinic. He has type 1 diabetes and had recently changed his insulin regimen on the basis of a raised HbA1C. Two weeks previously he had lost consciousness at a street party and required aid from the attending paramedics. The following week the police stopped him for cycling his bicycle erratically and aggressively, and since then he has had several other episodes of confusion. He is otherwise fit and well. He has a history of childhood epilepsy controlled with carbamazepine. He has not had a generalized seizure for 2 years. He is a non-smoker, does not drink alcohol and denied illicit drug use.

Examination is unremarkable. His blood pressure is 130/70 mmHg.

Blood results are as follows:

HbA1C	5.6%
Urinalysis	negative
ECG	normal sinus rhythm
Sodium	128 mmol/L
Potassium	3.5 mmol/L
Urea	6.0 mmol/L
Creatinine	87 μmol/L
Ca	2.5 mmol/L
Bicarbonate	24 mmol/L
Hb	13.2 g/cL
WCC	11.3 × 10⁹/L
Platelets	232 × 10⁹/L

What is the likely cause of his current symptoms?

1. Hypoglycaemia unawareness syndrome
2. Complex partial seizures
3. Syndrome of inappropriate antidiuretic hormone
4. Addison's disease
5. Adrenal insufficiency

Answer to Question 153 *is on page 382*

A 28-year-old male is sectioned and admitted to the psychiatric ward with a diagnosis of acute schizophrenia. Ten days later he becomes pyrexial and is unable to eat; his condition deteriorates over the subsequent 24 h and he becomes increasingly confused. On examination he has a temperature of 39.5°C, a pulse of 130/min, and blood pressure 145/90 mmHg. He has marked neck stiffness, normal fundi and symmetrically-increased tone in all four limbs with flexor plantars.

INVESTIGATIONS

Sodium	140 mmol/L
Potassium	4 µmol/L
Bicarbonate	28 mmol/L
Urea	5 mmol/L
Bilirubin	23 µmol/L
Alkaline phosphatase	120 iu/L
Aspartate aminotransferase	54 iu/L
Calcium	2.4 mmol/L
Creatinine kinase	980 iu/L
Glucose	4.3 mmol/L
Hb	12 g/dL
WBC	12×10^9/L
Platelets	230×10^9/L
Chest X-ray	normal
CT head	normal
Blood cultures	sterile
Urine dipstick	negative blood, negative protein
CSF	
Opening pressure	15 cm H_2O
Cell count	3 lymphocytes/mm^3
Protein	0.5 g/L
Glucose	3 mmol/L

What is the likely diagnosis?

1. Viral encephalitis
2. Bacterial meningitis
3. Acute schizophrenic episode
4. Neuroleptic malignant syndrome
5. Rhabdomyolysis secondary to underlying sepsis

Answer to Question 154 *is on page 383*

A 38-year-old primary school teacher is in casualty with a 6-month history of malaise and joint pains mainly affecting her hands, feet and ankles associated with mild stiffness in the mornings. There was no preceding viral illness. Her GP has prescribed non-steroidals and in the previous 2 months 20 mg of prednisolone, with little improvement.

Over the previous week she has had constant stiffness and swelling of the small joints of her hands and feet, particularly in the morning. For 48 h she has had a mild fever, back pain and progressive swelling of her left knee. Prior to this illness she was fit and well. Her father suffered from gout and diabetes, and her mother from hypothyroidism.

On examination she is clearly in pain and has great difficulty walking and undressing. She is pyrexial, has a temperature of 37.5°C, a pulse of 90/min, and blood pressure 110/70 mmHg. The small joints of her hands, wrists and feet are symmetrically swollen but not erythematous. She also has a very swollen large, red, and tender left knee with a lot of pain in the left calf.

INVESTIGATIONS

Haemoglobin	9.8 g/L	
WCC	15×10^9/L	neutrophils 11×10^9/L
Platelet count	600×10^9/L	
MCV	80 fL	
ESR	80 mm/h	
Urea and electrolytes	normal	
Liver function tests	normal	
C-reactive protein	360 mg/L	
Urine dipstick	trace of protein only	
ECG	sinus tachycardia	

a) What is the most important immediate diagnosis to exclude?
  1. Acute gout
  2. Septic arthritis of the left knee
  3. Infective endocarditis
  4. Ruptured left Baker's cyst
  5. Left deep vein thrombosis

b) What is the most likely underlying diagnosis?
  1. Polyarticular gout
  2. Rheumatoid arthritis
  3. Reiter's syndrome
  4. Systemic lupus erythematosus
  5. Adult Still's disease

Question continued overpage

c) The two most important investigations to perform are:
   1. Urine microscopy and culture
   2. Anti-cyclical citrillinated peptide antibody
   3. Serum urate
   4. Rheumatoid factor
   5. Aspiration of synovial fluid from left knee for microscopy and culture
   6. ANA
   7. Isotope bone scan
   8. Blood cultures
   9. Chest X-ray
   10. Urine microscopy and culture
   11. Serum ferritin
   12. ECHO

Answer to Question 155 *is on page 384*

An 80-year-old female is reviewed in the clinic in relation to the results of investigations for persistent low back pain and immobility. She is a lifelong smoker who also has chronic obstructive pulmonary disease which is usually controlled with home nebulizers, occasional courses of antibiotics and steroids. Although still mentally very alert, she is housebound and relies on meals on wheels.

Examination reveals a frail, elderly but orientated lady who has difficulty standing from the chair. She has tenderness over the lower spine.

INVESTIGATIONS

Sodium	140 mmol/L
Potassium	4.0 mmol/L
Urea	5.4 mmol/L
Creatinine	90 µmol/L
Ca	2.1 mmol/L
Phos	0.49 mmol/L
Albumin	40 g/L
ALP	218 iu/L
Bicarbonate	23 mmol/L
Other	

Pelvic X-ray: there is bone remocelling of the pelvis and loss of bone density.
Bone scan: multiple areas of increased activity.

What is the most likely cause of her back pain?

1. Hypoparathyroidism
2. Osteoarthritis
3. Osteomalacia
4. Osteoporosis secondary to steroid use
5. Post-menopausal osteoporosis
6. Myeloma
7. Fanconi syndrome
8. Paget's disease of the bone

Answer to Question 156 *is on page 385*

A 27-year-old female with type I diabetes attends the clinic for diabetic review. She initially presented at the age of 16 years in diabetic coma. She has had longstanding problems with compliance and erratically monitors her sugar levels. Over this period she had also had problems with recurrent cystitis.

On examination she is overweight. Cardiovascular, abdominal and respiratory systems are unremarkable. She has palpable peripheral pulses and no abdominal bruits. Her blood pressure is 120/80 mmHg and she is apyrexial.

INVESTIGATIONS

Glycosylated Hb	8.7%
Sodium	134 mmol/L
Potassium	3.4 mmol/L
Urea	6.4 mmol/L
Creatinine	108 µmol/L
Urinary albumin:creatinine ratio	2.5 mg/mmoL
Urine microscopy	No white cells, red cells, no organisms

Which treatment will best retard the progression of renal failure in the long term?

1. Tighter insulin control
2. Beta blocker
3. ACE inhibitor
4. Reduction in salt intake
5. Long-term antibiotic therapy to prevent recurrent urinary tract infections

Answer to Question 157 *is on page 387*

A 50-year-old, self-employed male had presented to the emergency department 3 weeks previously with chest tightness. He was told that his ECG showed no evidence of a myocardial infarct and on that basis decided to go home against medical advice. His wife has forced him to return. He has no other history aside from hypertension treated by his GP. Clinical examination is normal.

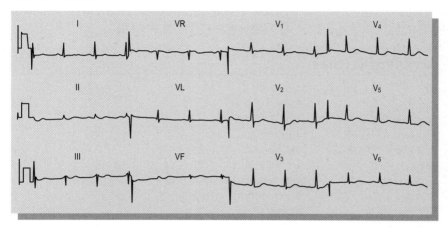

What is the likely diagnosis that accounted for his original presentation?

1. Pulmonary embolus
2. Pericarditis
3. Posterior myocardial infarction
4. Right bundle branch block
5. Right ventricular infarction

Answer to Question 158 *is on page 388*

A 40-year-old housewife presents to the OPD with a history of painful joints. Over the previous 2 months she had noticed particularly painful hands and a worsening of a rash on her face and arms when gardening outside. She had also noticed a raised rash on the back of her legs. She has a past history of hypothyroidism and takes thyroxine 100 mcg daily.

On examination she looks well. She has some tenderness over her wrists and elbow joints. She has a patchy erythematous scaling rash over her lower face and shoulders. Her blood pressure is 160/85 mmHg.

INVESTIGATIONS

Hb	12.2 g/dL
WCC	4.1 × 10⁹/L
Platelets	120 × 10⁹/L
Sodium	138 mmol/L
Potassium	4.3 mmol/L
Urea	6.1 mmol/L
Creatinine	140 µmol/L
Glucose	5.1 mmol/L
CRP	4 mmol/L
Urine dip	protein ++, blood +
	granular casts on urinary sediment

Miscellaneous

ANA	1:320 speckled pattern
Complement	low C3 and low C4
24-h protein	5.1 g/24 h

a) What is the most likely underlying diagnosis?
1. Cryoglobulinaemia
2. Polyarteritis nodosa
3. Nephrotic syndrome
4. Raynaud's disease
5. Systemic lupus erythematosus
6. Porphyria cutanea tarda
7. Rheumatic fever

b) What further investigation would help to monitor her disease?
1. Skin biopsy
2. Renal biopsy
3. Anti-double stranded DNA titres
4. Cryoglobulins
5. Anticardiolipin antibodies

A 30-year-old male is referred with fertility problems.

Examination reveals scanty axillary and pubic hair, soft testes, full visual fields and anosmia.

Investigation confirms a male karyotype. Testosterone, follicle-stimulating hormone and luteinising hormone concentrations are undetectable after gonadotrophin-releasing hormone is given intravenously. Thyroid-stimulating hormone, prolactin concentrations and a computed tomogram of the head are normal.

Which further test may give a diagnosis?

1. Serum transferrin and ferritin concentrations
2. Serum caeroplasmin levels
3. Glucose tolerance test
4. Testicular biopsy
5. Overnight dexamethasone suppression test

A 54-year-old office worker with type II diabetes mellitus is concerned that he should be on a lipid-lowering agent for his diabetes, having read a recent newspaper article. He has had diabetes for 8 years, is overweight and is a lifelong non-smoker. There is no family history of cardiac disease. He takes metformin 500 mg tds and is on no other medication.

Review of the notes reveals the following:

HbA1C	7.2%
Urine dip	negative
Blood pressure	140/80 mmHg
Total cholesterol	6.2 mmol/L
LDL	3.8 mmol/L
Renal function	normal

Using your evidence-based knowledge, how would you advise him on this issue?

1. Reassure that there is no need to currently prescribe a lipid-lowering agent but that you will arrange for dietary and lifestyle advice
2. Advise that you would need further evidence of raised lipid levels
3. Commence a statin
4. Commence a fibrate
5. Reassure and commence vitamin E

A 29-year-old single mother with a 4-month history of amenorrhoea and weight gain is referred by the GP. She has a history of anxiety episodes for which she had been prescribed an antidepressant 12 months previously. She also had a childhood history of epilepsy but has been fit free since then, although she does admit to periods associated with heavy alcohol binge-drinking where she has no recollection of whether or not she might have had seizures. Examination is unremarkable.

The GP encloses the following hormonal profile:

FSH	1.1 U/L	2–8
LH	12 U/L	6–13
Oestradiol	28 U/L	10–55
Testosterone	9.4 U/L 1–2	
Basal prolactin	5500 U/L	<390 mU/L

What is the most likely diagnosis?

1. Pituitary microadenoma
2. Secondary to medication
3. Pregnancy
4. Polycystic ovarian syndrome
5. Secondary to unwitnessed seizure activity

Answer to Question 162 *is on page 393*

A 55-year-old female is admitted by ambulance, with a widespread raised erythematous rash immediately after eating shellfish. She is acutely dyspnoeic with audible wheeze and a hoarse voice. She is still conscious. The paramedic team has already established IV access. Observations from the ambulance: pulse 110/min, blood pressure 80/60 mmHg, respiratory rate 28/min, O_2 saturation 90% on oxygen.

a) What would be your immediate management?
   1. Chlorpheneramine 10 mg slow IV
   2. Hydrocortisone 200 mg slow IV
   3. Adrenaline 1/10 000 solution 0.5 mL IV
   4. Adrenaline 1/1000 solution 0.5 ml IM
   5. IV fluid resuscitation and observe closely

b) How might you confirm the diagnosis?
   1. C1 inhibitor concentrate
   2. Measure serum mast cell tryptase
   3. Serum immunoglobulin levels
   4. Skin biopsy
   5. Rechallenge with shellfish

Answer to Question 163 *is on page 395*

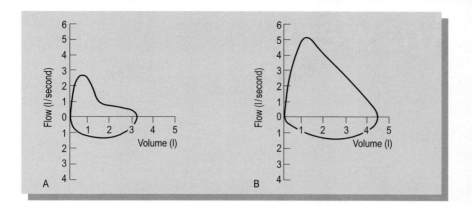

A 32-year-old non-smoker is admitted for investigation and treatment of severe shortness of breath. The following results are obtained:

Hb	14.3 g/dL
WCC	15.4 × 10^9/L
Neutrophils	74%
Lymphocytes	12%
Eosinophils	11%
PO^2	8.4 kPa
pCO^2	5.4 kPa
PEFR	80 L/s
Flow-volume loop A	

a) What diagnosis would account for flow-volume loop A?
 1. Intrathoracic obstruction
 2. Reversible obstructive airways disease
 3. Restrictive lung disease
 4. Extrathoracic obstruction
 5. Pneumonia

The patient's condition deteriorates over the next 12 h and he is subsequently electively ventilated via a cuffed endotracheal tube. He is weaned from the ventilator 4 weeks later. A flow-volume loop is performed 4 months later (B).

b) What diagnosis would account for flow-volume loop B?
 1. Pneumothorax
 2. Intrathoracic obstruction
 3. Tracheal stricture
 4. Vocal cord palsy
 5. Asthma

Answers

4. Acquired renal tubular acidosis.

This patient has developed acquired renal tubular acidosis secondary to the administration of amphotericin. He is hypokalaemic and the low bicarbonate is suggestive of a metabolic acidosis. In addition he also has a normal anion gap.

Anion gap = $\{[Na^+] + [K^+]\} - \{[Cl^-] + [HCO3^-]\} = 7\text{--}17 \text{ mmol/L}$

He had in fact been commenced on amphotericin B as part of a regimen for the treatment of neutropenic sepsis. The administration of amphotericin can be associated with causing a type I or distal renal tubular acidosis.

Causes of a hyperchloraemic normal anion gap metabolic acidosis
1. Renal tubular acidosis types I and II
2. Drugs: acetazolamide
3. Ureteric transplantation
4. Biliary or pancreatic fistulae
5. Severe diarrhoea

2. Carbon monoxide poisoning.

The blood gas results show a mild metabolic acidosis with a reduced pCO_2. Combined with the history, the most likely diagnosis is carbon monoxide poisoning. This patient has also had repeated episodes where she has been admitted and subsequently recovered; this can be a common but overlooked presentation of carbon monoxide poisoning.

- The diagnosis is made by direct measurement of the arterial carboxyhaemoglobin level.
- Pulse oximetry will often give a high reading of haemoglobin oxygenation in carbon monoxide poisoning as it cannot distinguish between oxyhaemoglobin and carboxyhaemoglobin. A direct measurement of oxygen saturation from a blood gas analyser is necessary. Carbon monoxide causes low arterial oxygen saturations in the presence of a well-maintained arterial PO_2.
- A carboxyhaemoglobin level of less than 10% is not normally associated with symptoms and 10–30% carboxyhaemoglobin may cause only headache and mild exertional dyspnoea.
- Patients may have a history of headaches, dizziness, convulsions, nausea and vomiting. On examination patients typically have a tachycardia, tachypnoea, cherry red lips; a cherry red spot at the macula and retinal haemorrhages can be present.
- Common sources of carbon monoxide are car exhaust fumes, improperly maintained and ventilated heating systems, smoke from all types of fire, and household gas (if supplies have not been converted to natural gas).
- Carbon monoxide has 240 times the affinity of oxygen for haemoglobin. The half-life of carboxyhaemoglobin in a patient breathing 21% oxygen is 180–300 min. This is shortened to 30–80 min by breathing 100% oxygen at 1 atm. It can be reduced further by the use of a hyperbaric oxygen chamber and evidence shows that this can reduce morbidity and mortality in patients with CO poisoning who suffer loss of consciousness. However, the relative accessibility of these devices may hinder their use but with CO poisoning and neurological sequelae, their use may be beneficial up to 24 h after presentation.

Answer to question 03

a) 2. Hereditary spherocytosis.

b) 4. Blood film.

Hereditary spherocytosis is the commonest inherited cause of a Coombs'-negative haemolytic anaemia. Inheritance is usually autosomal dominant and the defect is an abnormality in the main structural protein of the red cell membrane that is called spectrin.

The history suggestive of recurrent haemolysis and splenomegaly is compatible with this diagnosis. Haemolysis is also indicated by a reticulocytosis, absent haptoglobins and a raised bilirubin. A blood film would show microspherocytes and the diagnosis may be confirmed by demonstrating increased red cell osmotic fragility. A full family study should then be performed on the direct relatives of patients with this disorder. Splenectomy is usually performed in all cases, though it is usually delayed until 5 years of age because of the increased risk of infection (especially pneumococcal). Prophylactic daily penicillin post-splenectomy and pneumococcal and haemophilus vaccinations are recommended pre-splenectomy.

Spherocytes are red cells that have lost membrane without the equivalent loss of cytoplasm. They occur as a consequence of an inherited or acquired abnormality of the red cell cytoskeleton and membrane, making the red cell fragile and prone to haemolysis.

Causes of spherocytosis

Inherited
- Hereditary spherocytosis
- Haemolysis – warm and cold haemolytic anaemia
- Transfusion reactions
- Haemolytic disease of the newborn

Other
- Sepsis (Clostridium perfringens welchii)
- Fresh water drowning
- Zieves syndrome
- Bartonellosis
- Snake bites

Spherocytes can also be present on the blood film associated with other abnormally-shaped cells (poikocytes) in the following conditions
- Hyposplenism
- Sickle cell anaemia
- Micro-angiopathic haemolytic anaemia
- Mechanical haemolytic anaemia
- Homozygous hereditary elliptocytosis

a) 5. Urinalysis and βHCG levels.

b) 3. Carpal tunnel syndrome.

This patient is pregnant. The alkaline phosphatase (ALP) is commonly moderately elevated due to placental production of this enzyme. Pregnancy is an anabolic state, and hepatic synthesis of many proteins (e.g. C3 and C4) is enhanced. However, the plasma volume is also increased, resulting in a dilutional anaemia and hypoalbuminaemia. Hyperpigmentation in a butterfly distribution is a well-recognized complication of pregnancy.

The symptoms of carpal tunnel syndrome are common in pregnancy and may respond to simple splinting but surgical decompression under local anaesthetic is an option for severe cases.

Answer to question 05

a) 3. Hypoadrenalism.

b) 3. Short synacthen test.

Acute withdrawal of oral steroids has precipitated an adrenal crisis secondary to long-term steroid useage and subsequent adrenal suppression. The adrenals are unable to respond to stress. In secondary adrenal failure baseline cortisol level may be normal (>140 nmol/L) making a random level unhelpful.

Remember that an abnormal synacthen test will show a minimal response to adrenocorticotrophic hormone (ACTH) at 30 min with **a rise to a peak of less than 550 nmol/L or an increase of less than 250 nmol/L.**

Immediate management priorities would be to commence intravenous:
- fluid resuscitation- with IV normal saline
- hydrocortisone sodium succinate 100 mg IV stat

Answer to question 06

2. Falciparum malaria.

The most likely diagnosis is falciparum malaria with acute tubular necrosis. This man returned from a stay in Kenya and malaria is the commonest cause of fever in a patient returning to these shores from an endemic area.

The differential diagnosis, however, is obviously wide and includes other infections, multisystem diseases such as systemic lupus erythematosus (SLE), and malignancy, especially lymphoma.

The features suggesting malaria are:
1. An intermittent fever not responding to antibiotics, with a history of travel to a malaria region. The incubation period is normally 8–25 days; however, partial antimalaria prophylaxis and the non-specific features often result in considerable delays in presentation.
2. Frontal headaches, non-productive cough, myalgias and diffuse abdominal pains are typical of *Plasmodium falciparum*; chest pains and arthralgias are also recognized features. Malaria in the early stages may easily be confused with a viral illness.
3. Personality changes are the earliest signs of cerebral malaria. The lack of focal neurology, both on examination and on CT scan, and the normal CSF findings make other diagnoses less likely.
4. The severity of the normochromic normocytic anaemia suggests malaria rather than another infection. Both haemolysis and dyserythropoiesis contribute to the anaemia in malaria. Massive haemolysis leads to haemoglobinuria, 'blackwater' fever.
5. Renal failure. Acute tubular necrosis is the main cause of acute renal failure in falciparum malaria. Several mechanisms contribute: (i) intravascular haemolysis and haemoglobinuria, (ii) hypovolaemia and renal vasoconstriction, and (iii) blockage of small blood vessels. *Plasmodium malariae* and *Plasmodium falciparum* may cause a nephrotic syndrome, with evidence of immune complex deposition in the mesangium and glomerular basement membrane. A unique feature of falciparum malaria is that parasitized red blood corpuscles (RBCs) have an increased ability to stick to endothelium; this is related to protuberances on the RBC surface expressing a molecule similar to thrombospondin which binds to fibronectin. Sequestration and blockage of parasitized RBC in capillaries of brain and kidney play an important role in damage to these organs.

Thick and thin blood films should be obtained to identify RBC parasites. With an appropriate exposure history and fever, repeated examination of blood smears or even a therapeutic trial of antimalarial chemotherapy is required.

Intravenous quinine and fluids is indicated for severe malaria and for those who cannot swallow. IV quinine is given for 7 days followed by a single dose of pyrimethamine-sulfadoxine (Fansidar). Blood sugar levels should be checked before and during quinine treatment because patients are prone to hypoglycaemia both before and during treatment. In general it is always wise to seek advice from the local expert on tropical disease.

a) 3. Acute intermittent porphyria.

The combination of acute abdominal pain, vomiting, epilepsy and a predominant motor neuropathy suggest the diagnosis. This is further supported by the hyponatraemia, raised serum bilirubin and aspartate trans-aminase levels.

b) 4. Urine-δ-aminolaevulinic acid and urinary porphobilinogen.

Both should be greatly raised during the acute attack; levels are also raised during remission. The addition of Ehrlich's aldehyde reagent to the urine should result in a pink colour due to the presence of porphobilinogen. A similar result is also obtained if the urine contains urobilinogen. The addition of *n*-butanol distinguishes porphobilinogen, which is insoluble in *n*-butanol, unlike urobilinogen, which is soluble.

2. Inactive carrier.

This patient is an inactive carrier because he is HBsAg +. He has developed antibodies to the envelope antigen (antiHBe (+)). The viral load is low and he has had persistently normal ALT/AST levels.

Chronic **HBV infection** is a leading cause of chronic hepatitis, cirrhosis and hepatocellular carcinoma, and 15–40% of patients with chronic hepatitis B will develop serious hepatic complications during their lifetime.

Chronic HBV can be defined as the persistence of HBsAg in a patient's serum for more than 6 months. Carrier status of HBV can be further characterized with the following:

1. *Virological*: detection of HBeAg or anti HBeAg in the serum. The level of HBV replication can be determined by quantification of HBV DNA.
2. *Biochemical*: serum alanine aminotransferase (ALT) levels.
3. *Liver histology*: assessment of the grade of hepatic inflammation and the stage of fibrosis.

The most important criteria for determining the status of a patient with chronic hepatitis B	
Terms	Diagnostic criteria
Chronic hepatitis B	Serum HBsAg positive for longer than 6 months. HBeAg and anti HBeAg may be positive or negative[a] Persistent or intermittent elevation of ALT/AST levels Serum HBV DNA levels $>10^5$ copies/mL Liver biopsy showing significant inflammation (with a necroinflammatory score ≥4)
Inactive hepatitis B carrier	Serum HBsAg positivity longer than 6 months HBeAg (-); antiHBe (+). Persistently normal ALT/AST levels Serum HBV DNA $<10^5$ copies/mL Liver biopsy[b] showing absence of significant inflammation (necroinflammatory score ≤4)
Resolved hepatitis B	Serum HBsAg (-); anti-HBc (+), HBeAg (-) Normal serum ALT levels History of known acute or chronic hepatitis B Undetectable serum HBV DNA (hybridization assays)[c]

[a]Chronic HBsAg carriers with HBeAg are potentially highly infectious via the blood borne or sexual route. Chronic HBsAg carriers with anti-Hbe are less infectious
[b]A liver biopsy is optional
[c]HBV DNA may be detectable using sensitive polymerase chain reaction assays

Other notes

- Quantification of the HBV DNA is essential to determine the level of viral replication in a patient with chronic HBV replication.
- In addition to the history and physical examination, initial assessment should include virological markers, liver function tests, alpha fetoprotein levels (as a screen for hepatocellular carcinoma) and an ultrasound scan.
- If patients have an elevated ALT then they warrant a liver biopsy.
- Not all patients require treatment. The endpoint of treatment is to achieve inhibition of viral replication and remission of liver disease and this equates to a HBV DNA $<10^5$ copies/mL and seroconversion to anti–HBsAg.
- Interferon alpha (an immunomodulator) and Lamivudine (a reverse transcriptase inhibitor) are currently used. Lamvudine is more efficacious and associated with fewer side-effects.

Summary of hepatitis serology

HBsAg

Presents 6 weeks after infection and persists for 12 weeks. Persistence for greater than 6 months defines a chronic carrier. This is the best marker of current infection. If patients are negative then they are likely to be non-infectious. (With many years of a chronic infection it can become negative but antibodies to the core protein would still be detectable).

Anti HBs (antibody to HBsAg)

This is produced in the convalescent stage of infection and implies recovery. It can also arise as a result of immunization with hepatitis B vaccine.

HBeAg

If a patient is HBsAg + then this can be tested – if present it indicates a high infectivity. During the first years of chronic infection, patients are HBeAg and HBsAg +; later on they develop antibodies to HBeAg and infectivity declines. HBeAg can become negative as can HBsAg but antibodies to the core protein (Anti HBcAg) would remain positive. Persistence of HBeAg indicates continuing infectivity.

Anti HBeAg (antibody to HBeAg)

Anti HBeAg rises after an acute attack and indicates low infectivity. Its persisting presence indicates chronic infection. Patients with longstanding infection may not stay anti HBeAg + but they will stay anti HBcAg +.

Anti-HBcAg (antibody to HBcAg)

This antibody is produced after natural infection. The absence of anti HepBc effectively excludes past or current infection in that patient. IgM antibodies are high with acute infections and low with chronic disease. IgG antibodies with absent sAg indicate recovery from past infection, and with positive sAg ongoing infection.

a) 2. *Mycoplasma pneumoniae.*

The man has presented with an atypical pneumonia associated with hepatitis, erythema multiforme (note the history of target lesions) and cold agglutinins, and he has subsequently developed a myocarditis.

Extrapulmonary manifestations of *M. pneumoniae* occur in over 10% of cases, generally within 3 weeks of the respiratory symptoms. The most important complications in terms of morbidity and mortality are cardiac (myocarditis and pericarditis) and neurological (meningitis, meningoencephalitis, ascending paralysis, transverse myelitis, cranial nerve palsies, cerebellar ataxia and a poliomyelitis-like illness). Other extrapulmonary problems are more common and include rashes (25%), hepatitis, pancreatitis (rare), cold agglutinins (50%), haemolytic anaemia, bullous myringitis, thrombocytopenia, arthritis, and rarely, glomerulonephritis.

M. pneumoniae may be confirmed by isolating the organism from the respiratory system and mycoplasma serology. Culture is slow and not always available. A four-fold rise in antibody titre with a peak at 3–4 weeks suggests a recent infection. A rise in the cold agglutinin titre and the detection of specific IgM antibodies also suggest recent infection.

Clinically it is important to consider other atypical infections including legionnaire's disease, Q fever, psittacosis and viral infections (Coxsackie A and B and cytomegalovirus).

b) 4. Erythromycin.

Treatment of *M. pneumoniae* is with a macrolide or tetracycline. Early treatment probably decreases the frequency of extrapulmonary complications, many of which are autoimmune in origin.

Erythema multiforme is an eythematous disorder characterized by annular target lesions. Blistering can occur and involvement of the mucosa is common. The severest form is called the Stevens Johnson syndrome: This is associated with a high fever, anterior uveitis, pneumonia, polyarthritis and renal failure.

Common causes of erythema multiforme
- 50% idiopathic
- Infections: herpes simplex, *Mycoplasma, Streptococcus,* diphtheria, typhoid, orf
- Drugs: sulphonamides, barbiturates, sulphonyureas, penicillins, phenytoin
- Others: neoplasms, rheumatoid arthritis, systemic lupus erythematosus, ulcerative colitis

a) 3. Retained gastric antrum.

b) 4. At laparotomy.

These patients have a degree of hypergastrinaemia that results in recurrent peptic ulceration. The fall in serum gastrin levels during the secretin test in a patient who has undergone a partial gastrectomy is highly suggestive of a retained gastric antrum. In contrast the gastrin level in cases of a gastrin-secreting tumour (Zollinger-Ellison syndrome) rises during the secretin test. In normal individuals, gastrin levels fall during the test. Up to 80% of patients develop a varying degree of steatorrhoea following partial gastrectomy.

a) 1. Coeliac disease.

b) 2. Anti-tissue transglutaminase antibodies.

c) 4. Stomatocytes.

Coeliac disease is a lifelong inflammatory disease of the small intestine occurring in genetically susceptible individuals. It is closely associated with the extended haplotype HLA-B8, DR3, DQ2; it is rare in those parts of the world where this haplotype is uncommon. The west coast of Ireland has the highest prevalence with up to 1 in 300 affected individuals.

The peak diagnosis in adults is in the third decade. 80–90% have general lassitude, 75–80% have diarrhoea, 85% have asymptomatic iron/folate deficiency. 15–30% have vitamin D deficiency, and 10% have vitamin K deficiency. Rarer problems include reduced fertility, psychological disturbances or a neurological deficit resulting in ataxia. There is often a delay of several years before the diagnosis is made.

The haemoglobin level may be low, The MCV can be low (iron deficiency) or high (folate deficiency), or commonly in the normal range reflecting a mixed picture. B_{12} deficiency is often less marked than folate deficiency unless large parts of the bowel are involved.

Malabsorption of the fat-soluble vitamins A, D, E and K often leads to their respective deficiencies. Serum concentrations of calcium, alkaline phosphatase, vitamin D, and the prothrombin time (INR) are routinely measured. Patients with diarrhoea may become hypokalaemic. Serum magnesium concentrations may also be low in severe coeliac disease and, with hypocalcaemia, can lead to tetany. Serum albumin is often low.

Serological screening tests can be performed for antibodies to gliadin, IgA antibodies to reticulin and IgA antibodies to endomysium. The endomysial antibody is the most useful with a sensitivity and specificity of 90–95%. The antibody is directed towards tissue transglutaminase and is detected by ELISA with transglutaminase coated wells. Antibody markers are also useful in monitoring as their level falls with compliance to a gluten-free diet. (If patients are screened for the presence of coeliac disease they should also have immunoglobulin levels checked concurrently. Five percent of patients with coeliac disease have concurrent IgA deficiency.)

A small intestinal biopsy is mandatory to confirm the diagnosis and many will rebiopsy after 6 months on a gluten-free diet to confirm histological improvement. The characteristic histological changes in a small intestinal biopsy are loss of height, crypt hyperplasia, a chronic inflammatory cell infiltrate and lymphocytic infiltration of the epithelium.

Treatment requires strict adherence to a gluten-free diet. The risks of lymphoma are increased in patients who do not adhere to a gluten-free diet. In addition the risks of developing other autoimmune disorders such as diabetes mellitus are also increased.

Other notes
- Dermatitis herpetiformis complicates 2–5%. It may be treated with Dapsone (note the side-effects of Dapsone, which include a haemolytic anaemia if the patient is G6 PD deficient, and methaemoglobinaemia).
- Hyposplenism invariably develops in patients with coeliac disease. This is usually associated with a lymphocytosis and an elevated platelet count. Abnormal features characteristic on the blood film of a patient with hyposplenism include target cells, acanthocytes and Howell jolly bodies. Small numbers of Pappenheimer bodies, Heinz bodies and spherocytes may also be noted.

Summary of disorders and complications associated with coeliac disease
- Dermatitis herpetiformis
- Lymphoma T cell, small intestine
- Increased risk of adenocarcinoma of the gut, carcinoma of oropharynx
- Chronic ulcerative enteritis (presents as protein-losing enteropathy)
- Neurological disorders – neuropathy, cerebellar, epilepsy
- Autoimmune diseases, e.g. diabetes, Addison's disease
- IgA nephropathy

Differential diagnoses of the causes of subtotal villous atrophy
1. Infectious enteritis in children
2. Giardiasis
3. Lymphoma
4. Whipple's disease
5. Hypogammaglobulinaemia
6. Cow's milk protein intolerance

a) 2. *Legionella* pneumonia.

b) 2. Erythromycin.

3. Rifampicin.

This patient has presented with an acute febrile illness characterized by gastrointestinal and respiratory symptoms, unexplained confusion, mild hepatitis, hyponatraemia, hypocalcaemia and relative hypophosphataemia. The most likely diagnosis is ***Legionella* pneumonia.** *Legionella* infection accounts for 2–5% of community-acquired pneumonia. Infection with *M. pneumoniae* or an ornithosis may have similar clinical features but these are not offered as options here.

Legionella occurs sporadically or in epidemics. The natural habitat of *Legionella* species is fresh water; a wide temperature (5–65°C) and wide pH range (5.5–8.2) is acceptable. Water storage systems such as air-conditioning apparatus, cooling towers and hospital hot water supplies have all been implicated as sources in a variety of epidemics.

Legionnaires' disease typically affects people between 40 and 70 years. There is a high incidence among transplant and other immunosuppressed patients. Abdominal symptoms may dominate the clinical presentation, including pain, diarrhoea and distension; rarely, peritonitis and pancreatitis occur. An enlarged liver and abnormal liver function tests are common. The pneumonia is typically widespread and may heal with fibrosis. In addition to confusion and hallucinations, ataxia, peripheral neuropathy and memory defects may occur. Hyponatraemia, hypocalcaemia, hypophosphataemia and lymphopenia are commonly seen. Haematuria occurs commonly; renal failure is rare. Pericarditis, myocarditis and endocarditis are rare.

Investigations should include urine sent for legionella antigen, sputum for culture, serology for *Legionella*, *Mycoplasma*, and *Chlamydia*. A bronchoscopy may be required to obtain material for culture and microscopy (if the condition and pO_2 of the patient permit). Soluble antigen is secreted in the urine for 1–3 weeks during the acute pneumonia and tests to detect *Legionella* serogroup urinary antigen 1 have high specificity and sensitivity making this the most valuable clinical test for prompt diagnosis.

Macrolide antibiotics such as clarithromycin and erythromycin are first line agents of choice. In patients with severe infections who are deteriorating, rifampicin or a fluoroquinolone should be added. The prognosis is related to the patient's age, the severity of the pneumonia and the existence of any concomitant disease. Symptoms of poor memory and general irritability may persist for months following recovery. Chlorination and filtration of water supplies will eliminate the organism.

a) 4. Gonococcal arthritis.

b) 1. Intravenous ceftriaxone.

Neisseria gonococci are a frequent cause of septic arthritis in young people. Radiology of the joint is normal unless the condition is left untreated, when severe destruction can take place.

Gonorrhoea occurs in females as frequently as in males; however, affected females generally have fewer symptoms and may act as asymptomatic carriers. Pregnant and menstruating females are more prone to haematogenous spread from vaginal foci. Arthritis and a vesiculopustular rash are the commonest complications. Others include endocarditis, meningitis, myocarditis and hepatitis. A mild fever and leucocytosis, raised ESR and CRP accompany gonococcaemia. Tenosynovitis, particularly of the wrists, hands, feet or Achilles tendon, occurs in two-thirds of cases. Tenosynovitis (in this case, evident as pain in the dorsum of her hand on movement), a fever and one or two swollen joints in a young person strongly suggest the diagnosis.

Investigations aim to isolate the Gram-negative intracellular diplococci.

Culture positivity	
Site	Isolation rate
Genitourinary	80%
Synovial fluid	25-30%
Rectum	20%
Pharynx	10%
Blood	5%
Skin	<5%

Ciprofloxacin has been widely used but the incidence of resistance is increasing and many authorities would now use a third line cephalosporin as their agent of choice. Local microbiological guidelines should therefore be consulted.

Other notes:
- Perihepatitis: the FitzHugh–Curtis syndrome more frequently appears with *Chlamydia trachomatis* than *Neisseria gonorrhoea*. Patients present with right hypochondral pain which may be referred to the shoulder and may have a pleural effusion.

Answer to question 14

a) 1. De Quervains thyroiditis.

b) 2. Reduced uptake.

The most likely diagnosis is subacute or **De Quervains thyroiditis** which can present with thyrotoxicosis. Symptoms usually follow an upper respiratory tract infection. A goitre may develop which can be tender with pain referred up to the jaw.

The erythrocyte sedimentation rate is typically raised in cases of De Quervains thyroiditis.

The technetium thyroid uptake scan will show reduced uptake as opposed to the increased uptake seen with Grave's disease, or the patchy uptake seen with toxic multinodular goitre.

Glucocorticoids can be used to control symptoms. The thyroiditis is often self-limiting although occasionally patients can become hypothyroid as thyroid hormone is rapidly depleted. Carbimazole is therefore not often indicated.

Notes:

In thyrotoxicosis, thyroid hormones are elevated and the TSH is suppressed because of feedback inhibition. In some cases the T3 may be elevated in isolation (T3 thyrotoxicosis) but the TSH will be suppressed. Measuring the free T4 alone however is usually sufficient to make a diagnosis.

Note that rarely, a normal or slightly raised TSH level in the face of hyperthyroidism can be seen with a TSH producing pituitary adenoma.

Some of the most common symptoms and signs in thyrotoxicosis

Symptoms	Signs*
Hyperactivity, irritability, dysphoria	Tachycardia: AF in the elderly
Heat intolerance and sweating	Tremor
Palpitations	Goitre
Fatigue and Weakness	Warm moist skin
Weight loss and increased appetite	Muscle weakness and proximalmyopathy
Diarrhoea	Lid lag/retraction
Polyuria	Gynaecomastia
Oligomenorrhoea and loss of libido	

*Excludes signs of opthalmopathy and dermopathy specific for Graves disease

2. **Anorexia nervosa.**

This is the most common reason for weight loss in this age group.

A recurrence of her previous malignancy is possible but some other systemic features such as a fever may be expected.

Brucellosis could also be a consideration especially with the added risk of drinking unpasteurised milk while in Greece. A history of general lethargy and episodic fevers is typical for chronic brucellosis.

The diagnosis of **anorexia nervosa** is a clinical one, based on the following findings: considerable weight loss, specific psychopathology associated with guilt about eating, loss of control and a disturbed body image where the patient perceives herself as overweight.

- Patients diet excessively, exercise keenly and may have experienced a recent emotional upset.
- On examination the patient may have signs of extreme weight loss, blue-cold hands and feet, dry skin with downy hair over the nape of the neck, cheeks, forearms and legs, and a low pulse pressure is often observed.
- LH, FSH and oestradiol levels are abnormally low. In the male, plasma LH and testosterone levels are low and there is loss of sexual interest and potency. Other blood results are likely to be normal unless self-induced vomiting is associated with electrolyte abnormalities.
- The increased incidence in western society, and among higher social classes, suggest that the aetiology is related to culturally determined attitudes.
- The aims of treatment are to obtain the patient's confidence and a degree of cooperation, restore their weight to a healthy level, reduce residual disability and shorten the duration of the illness.

Other notes:
Brucellosis is a zoonosis caused by *Brucella melitensis, B. suis* or *B. abortus*, in decreasing order of frequency in humankind.

- The organism is a small Gram-negative coccobacillus which is an intracellular pathogen. Primary infection may be acute, chronic or subclinical.
- It may be contracted from milk or soft cheeses, tending animals and handling the carcasses of infected animals, and is an occupational disease of farmers and related professions.
- The bacillus enters across mucous membranes, is phagocytosed, reaches lymph nodes and there replicates. It is released when the cell is disrupted and reaches the liver and spleen.
- Chills, sweats, aches and pains, general lethargy and episodic fevers are typical. On examination there may be evidence of an arthritis, spinal tenderness, bursitis, splenomegaly, orchitis and meningo-encephalitis.

- Granulocytopenia may be the first clue to the diagnosis, and lymphocytosis can occur when it is chronic. The diagnosis is made either serologically or by isolation of the organism from blood cultures, bone marrow aspirate or pus.
- Treatment is with tetracycline if the condition is diagnosed early, otherwise streptomycin must be added. Doxycycline and rifampicin are also an effective therapeutic combination. Spontaneous resolution occurs after months without treatment; relapse is common and may occur within 2 months of treatment.

a) 3. Common variable immunodeficiency (CVID).

b) 5. Immunoglobulin levels.

CVID is an acquired antibody deficiency. B-cells are usually present but fail to produce IgG, IgA and occasionally IgM. The clues are: chronic childhood infections (mostly bacterial), chronic diarrhoea with *Giardia lamblia*, and low immunoglobulins (normal albumin but a low total protein). Chronic respiratory tract infections may lead to bronchiectasis (suggested by the examination findings in this patient), pulmonary fibrosis, cor pulomonale and early death. Twenty percent of patients develop a granulomatous reaction that is characterized by multiple tissue granuloma in the lymphoid tissue, liver, spleen and lungs. This is usually steroid responsive. There is also an increased incidence of autoimmune disease and malignancy. The possibility of a lymphoma should be considered if lymphadenopathy is a major feature. Patients can also develop a symmetrical large joint non-erosive arthritis but it is always important to consider the possibility of septic arthritis, (particularly *Mycoplasma*). Vitamin B_{12} deficiency and atrophic gastritis are not uncommonly seen in these patients.

Other notes

- *Cystic fibrosis* is an important differential to consider, particularly with the history of bronchiectasis, but the patient would be very unlikely to present at this age without other complications such as diabetes. The low immunoglobulin level also makes this unlikely.
- *Chronic granulomatous disease* is associated with an abnormality in neutrophil killing due to a defect in NADPH oxidase; this leads to impaired oxygen dependent killing and an increased incidence of infection with catylase positive organisms. Patients have chronic suppurative abscesses or granulomas affecting skin, lung, liver and lymph nodes, as well as osteomyelitis. They present in early or late childhood years. The condition is X-linked recessive in two-thirds of cases, making presentation in a female much less likely. The neutrophil respiratory burst pathway is assessed by the Nitroblue tetrazolium (NBT) test or by flow cytrometry. (Neutrophils fail to reduce the substances they have phagocytosed.)
- *Complement deficiences* C3, C1q cause increased susceptibilty to capsulated bacteria and immune complex disorders such as SLE. Deficiencies of C5–C9 cause susceptibility to disseminated neisserial infections.
- *The Chediak-Higashi syndrome* is a rare autosomal recessive disorder characterized by partial oculocutaneous albinism, frequent pyogenic infection, and the presence of abnormally large cytoplasmic granules in neutrophils and other cells. Death is usually in childhood or adolescence due to infection or lymphoproliferative disease. There is an impaired phagocyte response to chemoattractants and reduced killing of phagocytosed bacteria.

2. Beta-thalassaemia minor.

This is the characteristic picture of a moderate hypochromic microcytic blood picture with normal haemoglobin and iron stores.

The most likely diagnosis is **beta-thalassaemia minor**. The diagnosis is often made when a routine blood count reveals a microcytic hypochromic anaemia in an asymptomatic patient. A raised HbA2 >3.5% confirms the diagnosis.

Other notes
- *Haemoglobin H disease* – three alpha gene deletions leads to a moderately severe microcytic anaemia (7-11g/dL) and splenomegaly is common.
- *Latent iron deficiency* – the ferritin would usually be low. In this case the ferritin is normal. Iron deficiency may be masked by an acute phase response and the ferritin would therefore rise because it is an acute phase protein. In this patient the viscosity is normal making this unlikely.
- Iron deficiency is the commonest cause of a hypochromic microcytic anaemia.
- The differential diagnosis for a hypochromic microcytic anaemia also includes:
  - Iron deficiency
  - Anaemia of chronic disease
  - Sideroblastic anaemia
  - Alpha- and beta-thalassaemia trait.

Causes of sideroblastic anaemia
Causes of sideroblastic anaemia can be an inherited (usually X-linked recessive) or acquired.
Primary
- Myelodysplastic syndromes – termed 'refractory anaemia' with ring sideroblasts seen in the marrow, this is a primary acquired sideroblastic anaemia
- Occasionally with myeloproliferative disorders
Secondary
- Excess alcohol consumption
- Isoniazid, chloramphenicol
- Lead poisoning
- Connective tissue disorders
- Malignancy

There is an abnormal type of red cell production. A substantial proportion of erythroblasts contain a perinuclear ring of coarse iron-containing granules. These are described as ring sideroblasts. They may be seen on a bone marrow aspirate. The granules are iron-laden mitochondria. The blood film may be dysmorphic or show uniform hypochromia and microcytosis.

Anaemia of chronic disease

Anaemia of chronic disease is commonly due to:

- Chronic infections
- Neoplasia
- Rheumatoid arthritis
- Renal failure

It is primarily due to the under-production of red cells. There is also a reduction in the red cell lifespan. The red cells are most commonly normochromic and normocytic but in 30–35% of patients they are hypochromic and microcytic.

a) 4. **Extrinsic allergic alveolitis.**

b) 3. **An elevated lymphocyte count with CD8>CD4.**

Extrinsic allergic alveolitis (EAA) or Hypersensitivity pneumonitis is a condition in which the patient is hypersensitive to spores of thermophyllic actinomycetes in mouldy hay. The most important steps in assessing a patient suspected of having EAA are:

1. **A full occupational history:** to identify the causative antigen and confirm appropriate exposure
2. Pulmonary assessment: lung function tests including gas transfer
3. Thoracic imaging: chest X-ray and high-resolution CT thorax
4. Bronchoscopy and broncheolar lavage: useful for excluding any macroscopic abnormality and for assessing differential cell counts in lavage fluid. An elevated lymphocyte count with CD8>CD4 would be expected
5. Immunological: the demonstration of an IgG precipitin response to the organic dust*
6. Transbronchial or open lung biopsy.*

* Histological confirmation may not be required in cases where there is little diagnostic uncertainty.

Extrinsic allergic alveolitis (Hypersensitivity pneumonitis) refers to a group of conditions (farmer's lung, bird-fancier's lung, mushroom-worker's lung, etc) in which inhaled organic dusts trigger a hypersensitivity reaction.

- Although many of these conditions are associated with specific precipitins (antibodies to the presumed antigen), complement activation by immune complexes (type III hypersensitivity) is no longer thought to be the only or even the most important mechanism causing lung damage. Cell-mediated (type IV) hypersensitivity is probably the most important process. Histology shows extensive lymphocyte infiltration of the alveolar walls and, in more advanced cases, granuloma formation and lung fibrosis.
- The acute form of extrinsic allergic alveolitis presents as an influenza-like illness (malaise, myalgia, fever, headache) and breathlessness with a dry cough but no wheeze. The symptoms commence 3–9 h after exposure to the sensitizing antigen. A period of exposure (several weeks to months) is required before the first attacks are noticed.
- In the chronic form the symptoms are less dramatic and there is gradual onset of dyspnoea on exertion.
- The most consistent physical sign is fine crepitations heard throughout the lung. Clubbing is very unusual. Patients may present with lung fibrosis or cor pulmonale that may be difficult to distinguish from cryptogenic fibrosing alveolitis or sarcoid.
- In severe forms hypoxia may be profound and the chest X-ray shows a ground glass appearance, particularly in the lower and mid-zones.
- The fibrosis may be predominantly in the upper lobes and simulate the chest X-ray changes of tuberculosis.

- Lung function tests vary according to the severity of the disease and the duration of time since exposure. The most common findings are impaired CO gas transfer (decreased TLCO and KCO) with a restrictive ventilatory defect (FVC is diminished as much as FEV_1 or more so. Lung capacity is reduced but residual volume is increased suggesting a degree of air trapping.
- High resolution CT scans show characteristic changes, the most frequent being increased ground glass density of the lung parenchyma, air trapping on expiratory scans and irregular linear and reticular opacities due to fibrosis.
- Bronchoscopy or bronchiolar lavage typically shows an accumulation of lymphocytes with an increase in the CD8:CD4 ratio. This differs from cryptogenic fibrosing alveolitis, where polymorphs predominate.
- The finding of precipitating IgG antibodies is not diagnostic since such antibodies are found in healthy people who have had appropriate exposure. However, the majority of affected patients have precipitans and their absence makes extrinsic allergic alveolitis unlikely.
- Transbronchial or open-lung biopsy may be required if other procedures are not characteristic.
- Treatment is avoidance of the responsible antigen. Steroids may be useful in a severe acute extrinsic allergic alveolitis.

3. Squamous cell carcinoma.

Hypercalcaemia is commonly seen in patients with malignant disease. This is usually due to increased calcium release from bone, but in some instances, and in about 15% of squamous cell lung carcinomas, it is due to the production of parathyroid hormone-related protein and other factors by the tumour itself. This latter syndrome has been variously described as pseudohyperparathyroidism or humoral hypercalcaemia of malignancy, and may occur in the absence of skeletal metastases.

- The majority of patients with carcinoma and hypercalcaemia have overt radiographic or scintigraphic evidence for bone metastases. Furthermore, parathyroid hormone (PTH) levels will be low.
- Patients with myelomatosis and other haematological tumours associated with hypercalcaemia may show diffuse osteoporosis rather than the more characteristic punched-out lesions.
- In the absence of renal impairment, a plasma bicarbonate may be useful. In hyperparathyroidism, a metabolic acidosis is commonly found which is reflected by low plasma bicarbonate and a high plasma chloride, whereas in disorders where PTH secretion is depressed a metabolic alkalosis is to be expected. Moreover, in hypercalcaemia due to rapid bone destruction, alkalosis may be accentuated by the release of bicarbonate from bone. Patients with carcinoma also frequently have low serum values of albumin and phosphate due to cachexia.

Small cell cancer is very rarely associated with PTH-related protein production but may produce inappropriate antidiuretic hormone secretion causing hyponatraemia or ectopic ACTH production causing Cushing's syndrome.

Other tumours that may produce parathyroid hormone-related protein
- Bronchogenic non-small cell carcinoma
- Breast cancer
- Squamous carcinoma of the oesophagus
- Other malignant gastrointestinal tumours
- Renal cell carcinoma
- T- or B-cell lymphoma
- Hepatoma
- Melanoma

2. Isoniazid, rifampacin, pyrazinamide and ethambutol.

Immunocompromised patients may develop tuberculosis due to reactivation of previously latent disease or due to new infection. Culture should always be carried out and the type of organism identified but this should not delay the initiation of treatment.

The commonest respiratory symptom is cough with mucoid then purulent sputum, which is sometimes accompanied by haemoptysis. Breathlessness typically only presents when there is significant parenchymal damage or if a pleural effusion develops.

There may be general features of infection such as nocturnal fever, anorexia and malaise. Weight loss may be considerable – up to 10 kg.

The chest X-ray may show typical features and extent of disease. Posterior segments of the upper lobes are the most commonly affected. Parenchymal disease often leads to cavitation. Diagnosis requires bacteriological confirmation and three morning sputum specimens should be taken. If these cannot be obtained and tuberculosis is likely, then patients should undergo bronchoscopy and lavage. For pleural effusions, pleural biopsy and cytology for culture, protein and cytology should be undertaken.

Tuberculosis is treated with an initial phase using at least three drugs and a continuation phase using two drugs in fully sensitive cases:

The initial phase
The initial phase should be continued for 2 months.
- This is designed to reduce the bacterial load quickly and prevent the emergence of drug-resistant strains.
- Treatment of choice is isoniazid, rifampacin, pyrinazamide and ethambutol.
- Ethambutol **can be omitted** from the regimen if the patient is not immunocompromised, not previously been treated, and has not been in contact with possible multi-drug-resistant strains of tuberculosis. (If susceptibility results are not available, full treatment should be continued.)

Continuation phase
- Treatment should be continued for another 4 months.
- Streptomycin is rarely used in the UK; it can be used if resistance to isoniazid is established before treatment starts.
- The standard regimen may be used in pregnancy.
- Isoniazid, rifampacin and pyrinazamide are associated with liver toxicity. Hepatic function should be checked before drugs are started.
- Renal function should also be checked: streptomycin and ethambutol should be avoided in patients with renal impairment.
- Visual acuity should be checked before the commencement of ethambutol.
- Note that all cases of tuberculosis require notification.

3. Small bowel barium meal.

This patient has a macrocytic anaemia and the vitamin B_{12} level is low with a high/normal folate.

The most likely cause, given her history, is the previous abdominal radiotherapy, which can cause an enteritis with subsequent stricture formation. This can predispose to bacterial overgrowth and vitamin B_{12} is metabolized by bacteria but they synthesize folate. The most useful test will be a barium study. This will determine whether there are any structural abnormalities such as adhesions or loops caused by the radiotherapy. It may also help determine whether there is any terminal ileal disease (common causes include Crohn's disease, ileal tuberculosis or small bowel lymphoma).

Other tests may be used to confirm malabsorption:
- The 14^C xylose test relies on the ability of anaerobic bacteria to metabolize this compound, resulting in the formation of radioactive CO_2 that is exhaled from the lungs. This may be used to confirm malabsorption.
- The bile acid (glycine-labelled glycholate) breath test works on the same principles. It has a higher false negative rate and also requires the concomitant measurement of the labelled compound in the faeces.

Other notes
- The Schilling test would be abnormal **with or without** the addition of intrinsic factor. The Schilling test can correct with the administration of antibiotics for 5 days.
- A small bowel biopsy and culture may prove diagnostic of bacterial overgrowth but these are often cumbersome and difficult to perform, although they remain the gold standard in terms of diagnosis.
- Conditions leading to bacterial overgrowth:
  1. Chronic atrophic gastritis/pernicious anaemia
  2. Subtotal gastrectomy and gastrojejunostomy
  3. Jejunal diverticulae
  4. Intestinal fistulae – underlying causes include Crohn's disease, tuberculosis, lymphoma, radiation enteritis and colonic diverticulosis
  5. Motility disturbances: systemic sclerosis, intestinal pseudo-obstruction, diabetic autonomic neuropathy, abdominal radiotherapy, amyloidosis
  6. Radiation enteritis causing adhesions
  7. Achloridia
  8. Hypogammaglobulinaemia.
- **Causes of vitamin B_{12} deficiency include:**
  1. Nutritional: vegans
  2. Gastric: addisonian pernicious anaemia, congenital deficiency of intrinsic factor, gastrectomy (partial or total) and atrophic gastritis
  3. Intestinal: blind loop syndrome, ileal resection, Crohn's disease, tropical sprue, fish tapeworm, transcobalamin 11 deficiency
  4. Drugs: para-aminosalicylic acid, colchicine, alcohol, biguanides.

a) 6. Prothrombin time.

b) 2. Continue N-acetylcysteine infusions and monitor closely.

The prothrombin time expressed as an international normalized ratio (INR) provides an index of hepatic synthetic capacity that applies to both acute and chronic liver injuries – it provides an indirect measure of hepatic synthesis of the clotting factors I, II, V, VII, IX, and X. Other causes of a prolonged prothrombin time include vitamin K deficiency, warfarin therapy and acquired and congenital clotting factor deficiencies. The INR has prognostic value in both acute and chronic liver failure, regardless of the aetiology.

Measurements of the prothrombin time are most useful when monitoring patients during the course of acute liver failure. In the King's college analysis a rise in the INR from days 3 to 4 was associated with a 7% survival compared with a 79% survival in those whose INR fell at that time.

A low arterial pH (reflecting metabolic acidosis) is also of importance and the King's college guidelines are widely used to assess patients who may require liver transplantation. The following guidelines help to rapidly categorize patients at greatest risk of fulminant liver failure.

King's college criteria for transplantation in acute liver failure
Paracetamol cases:
- pH <7.3 (irrespective of grade of encephalopathy) or
- Prothrombin time >100 s and serum creatinine >300 if in grade III or IV coma

In non-paracetamol cases:
- Any three of the following irrespective of the grade of encephalopathy:

  1. Aetiology: non-A, non-B (indeterminate) hepatitis, halothane hepatitis, idiosyncratic drug reactions

  2. Age <10 or >40 years

  3. Jaundice to encephalopathy interval >7days

  4. Prothrombin time >50 s

  5. Serum bilirubin >300 μmol/L

From Devlin J, O'Grady J 1999 Indications for referral and assessment in adult liver transplantation: a clinical guideline. Gut (suppl 6):VI1–VI22

Other biochemical markers of liver function
The aminotransferase enzymes – aspartate aminotransferase (AST) alanine aminotransferase (ALT) are the most commonly used markers of hepatocyte necrosis. ALT is highly specific for the liver, but AST is located in the heart, brain, kidney and skeletal muscle and is therefore less specific for liver injury.

Serum alkaline phosphatase (ALP) is produced by a variety of sources including the liver, bone, leukocytes and the placenta. Levels increase in most types of liver injury and this is because bile acids induce alkaline phosphatase synthesis. Less than a three-fold increase is not specific for any particular type of liver injury. The highest concentrations occur with cholestatic injuries. Concentrations do not specify between intrahepatic and extrahepatic aetiologies and the specificity for the liver is poor: other conditions such as bone diseases, growth spurts or pregnancy can also increase serum values.

Serum gamma - glutamyltransferase (γGT) enzymes are located in a variety of tissues including the heart, brain, kidney, spleen and the billary ductile cells of the liver. The most use that can be gained from monitoring serum γGT is in the exclusion of bone disease as a cause of a raised ALP. The enzyme is also inducible by chronic alcohol use and by drugs such as phenytoin.

Free bilirubin is not water-soluble and must be bound to albumin. It is then taken to the liver where it is conjugated and excreted in the bile. The conjugated fraction is therefore also excreted in the urine. Mild-to-moderate unconjugated hyperbilirubinaemia is generally associated with haemolysis; inherited defects in hepatic uptake or conjugation can cause a similar pattern. When hepatic injury is present, the direct bilirubin fraction is typically at least 50% of the total serum value. Urine bilirubin is a more sensitive indicator of liver injury and this has prognostic value in patients with chronic failure. It has been shown to be less useful in acute hepatic decompensation.

Albumin is the major plasma protein synthesized in the human liver and is a clinically useful marker of hepatic synthetic function. It has a half-life of 20 days and is therefore not useful in acute hepatic injury.

Other notes
- Biochemical measurements provide a static assessment of the degree of liver injury but provide less evidence of the continued hepatic function. Caffeine is metabolized by the liver, and caffeine metabolites can be measured in the urine or via a breath test. This is not routinely performed and although it does provide some indication of hepatic function it is not useful as a marker of prognosis.

a) 4. Spinal osteomyelitis with spinal cord compression.

b) 1. Blood cultures.

   3. MRI scan of thoracic spine.

   6. CT guided biopsy of affected vertebrae.

There has been nerve root involvement resulting in a sensory level at T4 and evidence of both pyramidal weakness and dorsal column involvement. Rectal tone is often preserved until late in spinal cord compression.

Radiology shows destruction of T4 and T5 vertebrae. The main differential diagnosis is between a malignant and an infectious process. Involvement of two adjacent vertebrae and loss of the disc space strongly suggests infection rather than malignancy. Night sweats that resolved after antibiotic therapy are a further clue. The lack of an acute phase response and the normal white blood count do not favour malignancy. Spinal osteomyelitis may be associated with little systemic upset and he had, furthermore, received antibiotics. The change in bowel habit in this case is as a result of opiate analgesia.

Back pain which radiates in a dermatomal distribution suggests nerve root involvement and therefore a disease process which involves the epidural space. The radiological appearance may lag behind the clinical disease by weeks or months.

The treatment for spinal osteomyelitis is intravenous antibiotics for 6 weeks, until the CRP normalises followed by oral antibiotics for 6–12 weeks. Accurate microbiological diagnosis is essential and may be obtained by guided biopsy if surgery is not required for spinal decompression.

The main organisms implicated in spinal osteomyelitis are *Staphylococcus aureus* (60%), enterobacteria (30%), acid-fast bacilli, *Brucella*, *Haemophilus influenzae*, *Nocardia*, *Candida*, and *Treponema pallidum*. Organisms usually spread via the blood stream but direct invasion may occur, e.g. from a pharyngeal abscess. Co-existing endocarditis should always be considered and an isotope bone scan will exclude other osseous lesions.

A neurosurgical opinion should be sought early as the prognosis is related to the speed of diagnosis, and surgical decompression must be undertaken early if it is to be successful. There are two principal mechanisms causing neurological damage: (i) the formation of an epidural abscess with a mass effect, and (ii) thrombosis of the spinal arteries.

1. **Send her blood sample to the nearest virology lab. If she has antibodies she is immune and no further action need be taken.**

If she is less then 20 weeks pregnant, there is a 1% risk that if she develops chickenpox, her baby could develop varicella syndrome. This is characterized by hypoplasia of the bone and muscle, rudimentary digits and skin scarring.

If she is more then 20 weeks pregnant there is no appreciable risk to the fetus.

If the mother is sure that she has had chickenpox previously then no further action is required. If she is not sure or she has no history of chickenpox then a sample can be tested for antibodies for varicella zoster virus. If she is antibody positive then no further action need be taken.

If she has no antibodies then the recommendation is to treat with Zoster immune globulin. This must be given **within 10 days** of contact and should reduce the severity of infection.

Ten percent of maternal varicella infections may be complicated by varicella pneumonia which has an appreciable mortality. Those pregnant women who develop varicella should also receive full dose aciclovir.

*Note: if the patient had been in contact with a member of her own family with chickenpox then she may well have had exposure to the virus for at least 48 h before the rash appears and therefore, in cases of doubt where there may not be enough time to test her antibodies, treatment with Zoster immune globulin is recommended prior to the antibody result.

3. Allopurinol.

This patient has sickle cell anaemia: She is therefore homozygous for HbS (the abnormality is due to substitution of valine for glutamic acid in position 6 of the beta chain). The cells can sickle at oxygen tensions usually found in the blood.

Sickled erythrocytes have an increased mechanical fragility and a shortened survival, which leads to a chronic haemolytic anaemia. When cells become irreversibly sickled they can form aggregates and as the viscosity of the blood increases this leads to vascular stasis, local hypoxia and further sickling: vaso-occlusion then leads to tissue infarction.

The haemoglobin is typically 6–9 g/dL; sickle cells and target cells occur in the peripheral blood, and haemoglobin electrophoresis is characterized by HbSS and no HbA with variable amounts of HbF (larger amounts are associated with milder symptoms). Screening tests are positive when the blood is deoxygenated.

Symptoms of anaemia are often mild in relation to the haemoglobin as the oxygen dissociation curve is shifted to the right, facilitating oxygen unloading. Symptoms vary greatly and some patients experience few crises whilst others have recurrent crises that may be painful, haemolytic, visceral (can lead to stroke) or aplastic (may be precipitated by low folic acid levels or parvovirus infection). Other complications include leg ulcers, hyposplenism, priapism, proliferative retinopathy, papillary necrosis, and nephrogenic diabetes insipidus. In children a painful dactylitis can lead to the hand–foot syndrome

Chief among the clinical features of sickle disease are acute episodes of severe pain in the chest, back, abdomen or extremities. Multiple areas are often involved simultaneously and symmetrical involvement of the extremities is common. The episodes can last for days or even weeks.

The **acute chest syndrome,** a frequent and sometimes fatal complication of sickle cell disease, affects about 40% of all people with sickle cell anemia. It is most common but least severe in children, can occur postoperatively, and when recurrent, can lead to chronic respiratory insufficiency. Its cardinal features are fever, pleuritic chest pain, referred abdominal pain, cough, lung infiltrates and hypoxia. There is often a prodromal illness.

Priorities in the management of the acute chest syndrome are to give effective oxygenation (up to 15% require intubation). Analgesia, usually in the form of intravenous opiates, is often required. Broad spectrum intravenous antibiotics should be commenced. Red blood cell transfusions appear to be as effective as exchange transfusions initially. Early specialist referral is mandatory.

High haemoglobin F concentrations reduce the severity of sickle cell disease.

Hydroxyurea increases the number of erythroblasts that produce haemoglobin F. Patients with more than three crises per year who take hydroxyurea have fewer episodes of acute chest pain syndrome and require fewer blood transfusions.

In contrast, patients with **sickle-cell trait** are heterozygous for HbS (having one gene for HbA and one for HbS, their cells contain beween 20–40% HbS).

They do not have cellular concentrations of HbS that are high enough for sickling under most conditions. They are usually haematologically normal and usually asymptomatic. Spontaneous haematuria can occur and renal papillary necrosis occurs rarely. It is possible for individuals to suffer vaso-occlusive episodes under conditions of unusual anoxia such as in unpressurized aircraft and occasionally under anaesthesia.

The sickle-cell trait causes no haematological changes and is diagnosed by the finding of a positive sickling test together with haemoglobins A and S on electrophoresis. Sickle-cell anaemia is diagnosed by the finding of a variable degree of anaemia, an elevated reticulocyte count, sickled erythrocytes on the peripheral blood film, a positive sickling test, and a haemoglobin electrophoretic pattern characterized by the absence of haemoglobin A and a preponderance of haemoglobin S with a variable amount of haemoglobin F. The diagnosis is confirmed by finding the sickle-cell trait in both parents.

Other notes
- Allopurinol inhibits xanthine oxidase. This enzyme converts xanthine and hypoxanthine to uric acid. Patients excrete less uric acid and more xanthine and hypoxanthine in the urine. Allopurinol is indicated for the treatment of recurrent gout.

> **2. Barium follow through may show fistulas and skip lesions.**

It is most likely that this patient is presenting with inflammatory bowel disease (IBD) – the major types being ulcerative colitis (UC) and Crohn's disease (CD). He has a typical history of abdominal pain, diarrhoea, rectal ulceration, erythema nodosum and sacroileitis. This history is more suggestive of Crohn's disease.

IBD is an idiopathic and chronic intestinal inflammation. The peak age of onset is between 15 and 30 years with a second peak between 60 and 80 years. The effects of cigarette smoking are different in UC and CD. Smoking reduces the risk of developing UC but increases the chance of developing CD. There is an increased family risk if a first-degree relative has IBD.

Key clinical features of Crohn's disease and ulcerative colitis
Crohn's disease can affect any part of the gastrointestinal tract from the mouth to the anus, but clinically rectal sparing is common.
- It tends to present with a history of right lower quadrant pain and diarrhoea. Weight loss associated with a low-grade fever is common. An inflammatory mass of inflamed bowel and mesentery may be palpable. Fistulas, fissures and abscesses may also develop.
- The process is transmural and is characterized endoscopically by small superficial ulcers or more active stellate lesions leaving islands of histologically normal tissue leading to the characteristic 'cobblestoning' appearance.

Ulcerative colitis extends proximally and in continuity from the rectum.
- It tends to present with diarrhoea, rectal bleeding, tenesmus, passage of mucus and crampy abdominal pain. Patients may have a tender anal canal and blood on rectal examination. Complications include a toxic colitis and toxic megacolon.
- It is a mucosal disease. Endoscopically the mucosa appears granular and friable and there may be spontaneous bleeding and ulceration. Single contrast barium enema typically shows fine mucosal granularity. Deep ulcerations can appear as collar button ulcers indicating mucosal penetration. The bowel wall is thickened and oedematous.

Extraintestinal manifestations of IBD affect up to a third of patients
Skin
- Erythema nodusum occurs in up to 15% of patients and is more common in CD. Pyoderma gangrenosum is seen in 1–12% of UC patients and less commonly in CD.
- Perianal skin tags are found in 75–80% of patients with CD.
- Oral mucosal lesions are commonly seen in CD and include apthous stomatitis and cobblestone lesions of the buccal mucosa.

Joints
- An asymmetrical, polyarticular migratory peripheral arthritis occurs in 15–20% of patients with IBD, is more common in CD and correlates

with bowel activity. It most often affects the large joints of upper and lower extremities.

- An asymmetrical sacroileitis occurs in 15–20%, again more commonly in CD. Sixty precent of these patients are HLA B27 +. The activity seems unrelated to bowel activity and does not improve with steroids. It often affects the spine and pelvis, and produces symptoms of low back and buttock pain and morning stiffness.

Ocular

- The most common symptoms are conjunctivitis, anterior uveitis and episcleritis. Uveitis is associated with both UC and CD colitis.

Hepatobiliary

- Primary sclerosing cholangitis (PSC) is characterized by intrahepatic and extrahepatic bile duct inflammation and fibrosis; this leads to chronic cholestasis and hepatic failure. A small proportion of patients with IBD have PSC but 75% of patients with PSC have ulcerative colitis. The diagnosis is made with ERCP which shows multiple bile duct strictures between normal segments.

Other notes

Infliximab is a chimeric human-murine monoclonal antibody that binds with high affinity to tumour necrosis factor alpha (TNF-α).

The over expression of TNF-α plays a pivotal role in the pathogenesis of Crohn's disease.

It is currently licensed for:

- Treatment of severe, active Crohn's disease in patients who have not responded to/or are unable to take corticosteroid and other immunomodulating agents such as azathioprine, 6 mercaptopurine or methotrexate
- Fistulating disease for which conservative or surgical treatment has failed or is inappropriate.

a) 1. Klinefelter's syndrome.

b) 4. Buccal smear.

Klinefelter's syndrome is the commonest cause of male hypogonadism. It is a developmental disorder of the testis that results from the presence of an extra X chromosome. The most common karyotype is 47 XXY.

Patients are sterile and have small firm testes. Males may be fully virilized and present with infertility or they may fail to reach sexual maturation. Patients may also have gynaecomastia, tall stature, learning difficulties and autoimmune endocrinopathies.

Levels of plasma follicle stimulating hormone (FSH) and luteinising hormone (LH) are high. The plasma testosterone is usually half the normal value.
The mainstay of treatment for the hypogonadal male is androgen replacement.

This patient is also likely to be osteoporotic as a result of testosterone deficiency and therefore should be commenced on calcium and vitamin D supplements and monitored with bone densitrometry scanning. For severe osteoporosis, biphosphonates remain an additional option.

Other notes
- *Kallmann's syndrome* is characterized by a family history (X-linked or autosomal) of hypogonadism and other stigmata, including anosmia or hyposmia (defective smell sense), red-green colour blindness, nerve deafness, and cleft-lip or palate. This is a hypogonadotrophic condition – levels of FSH and LH will therefore be low. It is caused by a defect in embryonic migration of GnRH-secreting neurons from their site of origin in the nose. They are therefore unable to reach the hypothalamus, from where their axons normally gain access to the portal circulation. The same migratory defect affects the olfactory neurons in the nose, resulting in aplasia of the olfactory bulb.
- *Noonan's syndrome* is an autosomal dominant condition that can occur in both sexes; it is characterized by a webbed neck, short stature and congenital heart disease (pulmonary stenosis) but patients have a normal karyotype and normal gonads.
- *Turner's syndrome* (gonadal dysgenesis) is characterized by primary amenorrhoea, sexual infantilism and short stature. About half have a 45, X karyotype and others have a mosaicism or structurally abnormal X chromosome. Other characteristic abnormalities involve the skeleton and connective tissue and include: lymphoedema of the hands and feet, webbing of the neck, low hairline, redundant skin folds, and a shield-like chest with widely spaced nipples. Short fourth metacarpals are present in half and 10–20% have coarctation of the aorta. The external genitalia are unambiguously female but remain immature, and there is no breast

development unless exogenous oestrogen is given. The fallopian tubes and uterus are immature, and bilateral streak gonads are present in the broad ligaments.

- *Marfan's syndrome* is an autosomal dominant condition characterized by, amongst other features, long thin extremities, joint laxity, lens dislocation and aortic root aneurysms. Most patients are heterozygous for mutations in a gene on chromosome 15 that encodes the fibrillin glycoprotein, which is a major component of elastin-associated microfibrils; these microfibrils are abundant in large blood vessels and the suspensory ligament of the lens.

5. **Pamidronate is effective in cases of hypercalcaemia associated with malignancy.**

Malignancy is the commonest cause of hypercalcaemia in hospitalized patients. Overall, hypercalcaemia occurs in approximately 5% of malignancies and is commonest with breast and lung lesions. Prostatic carcinoma commonly metastasises to bone, but lesions that are osteosclerotic and hypercalcaemia are rare. In the majority of cases, hypercalcaemia occurs in the setting of disseminated disease; only rarely is it the presenting feature of malignancy.

Symptoms of hypercalcaemia associated with malignancy include nausea, vomiting, thirst, polyuria, impaired renal function, constipation, abdominal pain and muscular weakness. Humoral hypercalcemia of malignancy should not be a consideration when the parathyroid hormone level is high, because the hypercalcaemic agent in this condition, parathyroid hormone-related protein, is not detected by the immunoradiometric assay for parathyroid hormone. Such patients also often have a hypochloraemic metabolic alkalosis which contrasts with the hyperchloraemic metabolic acidosis of primary hyperparathyroidism.

Symptoms of hypercalcaemia may be improved by simply rehydrating the patient. Once this has been achieved frusemide may be used to increase urinary calcium excretion. Thiazides are contraindicated, since they can cause hypercalcaemia, and increased PTH per se.

Bisphosphonates given intravenously (e.g. pamidronate) are also commonly used to reduce the hypercalcaemia of malignancy. They are also highly effective at reducing malignancy-associated bone pain.

Differential diagnoses of hypercalcaemia
- Malignancy
- Hyperparathyroidism – primary or tertiary
- Sarcoidosis
- Multiple myeloma
- Vitamin D intoxication
- Immobilized cases of Paget's
- Thyrotoxicosis
- Adrenal failure
- Milk alkali syndrome
- Phaeochromocytoma
- Thiazide diuretics (increase renal tubular calcium reabsorption)
- Artefactual causes, e.g. venous stasis
- Familial hypocalciuric hypercalcaemia

a) 5. C1-esterase inhibitor deficiency.

b) 6. Measure C4 level.

c) 2. Danazol.

C1 is a serine protease inhibitor that is involved primarily in the regulation of the early components of the 'classic' complement cascade; it also has a regulatory role in other pathways.

Insufficient normal C1 inhibitor leads to uncontrolled activation of the classical complement pathway with subsequent reduction of serum C4 and C2 concentrations.

Deficiency results in recurrent oedema typically affecting the face, larynx and gastrointestinal mucosa, which can lead to severe abdominal pain.

C1 inhibitor deficiency can be inherited or acquired. The hereditary form is autosomal dominant. Eighty five precent of patients have low levels of C1 inhibitor at presentation; the remaining 15% have abnormal C1 inhibitor function but the levels may be normal.

A low C4 level (with a normal C3) is the hallmark of hereditary and functional C1 inhibitor deficiency. Conversely, a normal C4 effectively excludes the diagnosis.

Severe episodes can be treated with C1 inhibitor concentrate. If this is not available, fresh frozen plasma may be given.

Danazol has been used for cases of hereditary angioedema associated with low C1 inhibitor concentrations. However, long-term danazol use has been associated with the development of hepatocellular adenomas.

Answer to question 30

a) 3. Restrictive lung defect with reduced gas transfer.

b) 1. High resolution CT thorax.

c) 2. Idiopathic pulmonary fibrosis.

The most likely diagnosis is **idiopathic pulmonary fibrosis** (cryptogenic fibrosing alveolitis). This is characterized by inflammation and fibrosis of the pulmonary peripheral air spaces and interstitium. It is most common in the 5th and 6th decades of life.

Key clinical features include the presence of clubbing in 70–80% and the characteristic fine to mid end-inspiratory crackles. The chest radiograph shows small lung volumes, and peripheral and basal reticulonodular shadowing. Lung function tests show a restrictive ventilatory defect with reduced gas transfer. HRCT will confidently provide the diagnosis in 90% of cases:

- In typical cases where there are characteristic CT findings then further diagnostic testing may not be necessary.
- If there is diagnostic uncertainty then further investigations such as broncheolar lavage and transbronchial lung biopsy may be undertaken which may provide a diagnosis in conditions such as sarcoidosis. Video-assisted lung biopsy may be required if diagnostic uncertainty remains.

The treatment of CFA can be guided by the CT findings and rate of progression of the disease. Treatment is recommended for the 'ground glass' appearances on CT scanning. Steroids are most commonly used, with the addition of azathioprine as a steroid-sparing agent.

a) 3. Chondrocalcinosis.

b) 3. Haemochromatosis.

Haemochromatosis is a common autosomal recessive inborn error of metabolism that affects the Caucasian population with a prevalence of between 1 in 200 and 1 in 500 and with an even higher prevalence in the Irish population. Males are affected more commonly than females and usually present in the 4th–6th decades.

Classic hereditary haemochromatosis is associated with a mutation of the haemochromatosis (HFE) gene on the short arm of chromosome 6; most cases are due to a single base change in the HFE protein at position 282 (C282Y) but there are other rarer genotypic and phenotypic variations. A positive iron balance is caused by its inappropriate absorption by the small intestine leading to iron deposition in the body tissues.

The classic triad of (i) diabetes, (ii) hepatomegaly and (iii) the slate-grey skin pigment (due to increased melanin deposition) may be accompanied by hypogonadotrophic hypogonadism, chondrocalcinosis, dilated cardiomyopathy, weakness and weight loss.

Increasing transferrin saturation values are the earliest biochemical hallmark.
The diagnosis may be confirmed by:
- Measuring the serum iron and ferritin concentrations: a fasting serum transferrin saturation greater than 45% and an elevated ferritin level should prompt investigation of the underlying phenotype.

Other appropriate tests include:
- A blood glucose level which will be elevated with the development of diabetes
- Gonadotrophin and testosterone levels – low with hypoganodotrophic hypoganadism
- A liver biopsy – this will show iron overload and the degree of hepatic damage
- A desferrioxamine infusion will show increased urine iron excretion
- X-rays of affected joints may show evidence of chondrocalcinosis.

The most commonly affected organs and their clinical features in patients with haemochromatosis		
Organ	Pathological change	Details
Liver	Cirrhosis	Hepatomegaly is present in 95% of symptomatic patients. Hepatocellular carcinoma occurs in 30% of cirrotics and is the most common cause of death
Pancreas	Diabetes	Occurs in about 65% of patients
Joints	Arthritis	Present in up to half of patients, usually occurs after the age of 50 years. The characteristic feature is chondrocalcinosis. The joints of the hands and the 2nd and 3rd metacarpophalangeal joints are the most commonly affected. A progressive polyarthritis involving the wrists, hips, ankles and knees may develop. Acute attacks of synovitis may be associated with depostion of calcium pyrophosphate (chondrocalcinosis or pseudogout)
Heart	Cardiomyopathy	The most common manifestation is congestive cardiac failure. The heart is diffusely enlarged and may be misdiagnosed as an idiopathic cardiomyopathy
Pituitary	Hypogonadotrophic hypogonadism	Occurs in both sexes and may be the presenting feature. Manifestations include loss of libido, impotence, amenhorrhoea, testicular atrophy, gynaecomastia and sparse body hair. Adrenal insufficiency, hypothyroidism and hypoparathyroidism may also occur

2. Transjugular intrahepatic stent shunt insertion.

Transjugular intrahepatic stent shunt (TIPSS) insertion is a radiological procedure that creates a communication between the portal and systemic circulation through the liver parenchyma. The tract is kept open with a stent and this lowers portal pressure and the risk of rebleeding.

It is the treatment of choice in cases of uncontrolled bleeding and in cases where rescue treatment is required for those who have failed endoscopic therapy. Insertion of TIPSSs, however, can be complicated by encephalopathy in 20% of patients and the gradual development of shunt insufficiency.

The acute management of variceal bleeding should centre initially on adequate resuscitation and airway protection to prevent aspiration.

Early endoscopy is recommended for variceal band ligation or sclerotherapy. Band ligation appears to have a stronger evidence base in this setting and is associated with fewer complications such as ulceration.

Glypressin has a systemic vasoconstricting and portal hypotensive effect and can be given if endoscopy is delayed or not readily available. Octreotide is a somatostatin analogue that can also be used in this respect.

Balloon tamponade is a highly effective procedure that arrests bleeding in 90% of cases, although rebleeding occurs in 50% when the balloon is deflated. This form of treatment is potentially life saving but is a temporary measure only.

a) 3. McArdle's disease.

b) 4. Muscle phosphorylase levels.

McArdle's disease is a glycogen storage disorder that occurs due to a genetic deficiency of muscle phosphorylase.

- This condition may remain unrecognized until early adulthood and then frequently presents with painful muscle cramps after exercise. Affected patients are not infrequently labelled as having a functional disorder, or 'chronic fatigue' syndrome.
- Inheritance is autosomal recessive.
- No rise in venous blood lactate is detected on exertion in these patients. The muscle biopsy will show an elevated concentration of glycogen and a deficiency in muscle phosphorylase.

Other notes

- *Von Gierke's disease (glucose 6 phosphatase deficiency)* is characterized by recurrent hypoglycaemia, hepatomegaly, short stature, delayed puberty, bleeding diathesis and hepatic adenomas, associated with increased serum lactate.

2. IV phentolamine.

This patient is having a hypertensive crisis due to massive catecholamine release by her phaeochromocytoma.

Phentolamine is a non-selective alpha adrenoceptor blocker. The dose for a hypertensive crisis due to a phaechromocytoma is 5–10 mg IV.
- Alpha blockade controls the blood pressure chiefly by abolishing peripheral vasonconstriction. In addition to alpha adrenoceptor block it also has direct vasodilator and cardiac inotropic actions.
- A beta blocker (such as propanolol) should not be given alone because the uncontrolled alpha adrenoceptor vasopressor effects are left unchecked without the peripheral beta adrenoceptor vasodilator action.
- Labetolol may also be used – this is a combined alpha and beta adrenoceptor blocking agent.
- The most commonly used treatment, however, to provide longer-term irreversible alpha blockade is phenoxybenzamine.
- Hydralazine is a centrally acting vasodilator that may be used in accelerated hypertension to reduce the blood pressure; the maximum effect is seen over 10–80 min.

Phaeochromocytomas are rare tumours of neuroectodermal origin that secrete catecholamines (adrenaline (epinephrine), noradrenaline (norepinephrine) and rarely dopamine).
- They are most commonly found in the adrenal medulla but can occur anywhere in the sympathetic nervous system.
- In adults they are most common in the 4th–5th decades.
- 10% are bilateral, 10% extra-adrenal, 10% familial and 10% malignant.
- Symptoms are dependent on the amount of catecholamine release and this often does not relate to the size of the tumour.
- The majority of patients present with dramatic paroxysms of hypertension associated with severe headaches, perspiration and palpitations. Between spells and up to time intervals of over 1 year, patients can be asymptomatic with a normal blood pressure. Fewer then 10% will have no such symptoms and presentation may be non-specific.
- Bilateral phaeochromocytoma occurs with greater frequency in patients with neurofibramatosis and von Hippel–Lindau disease. They also form part of MEN II syndromes where there is an association with medullary thyroid carcinoma and hyperparathyroidism and in MEN2b – also a marfanoid habitus with mucosal neuromas.
- Biochemical confirmation is with 24-h urine catecholamine (urinary vanillylmandelic acid (VMA)) or by the less commonly used but more sensitive metanephrine collections. Plasma catecholamines can be measured but they have a high false–positive rate.

- CT scanning is the most widely used modality for localization of the tumour.
- MR imaging may also be used if contrast media is contraindicated.
- If there are difficulties then scintigraphic localization with 131 – I metaiodobenzylguanidine (MIBG) may be used.
- Surgical excision is mandatory and patients require an alpha blocking agent such as phenoxybenzamine. (Unopposed alpha 1 vasoconstriction can cause significant hypertension, cardiac ischaemia and pulmonary oedema.) Beta adrenoceptor blockade is then also required to control tachycardia.

4. Add rosiglitazone in combination with metformin.

Rosiglitazone is a thiazolidione – a peroxisome proliferator activated receptor – gamma agonist (PPARG). It acts by reducing the body's resistance to the action of insulin.

Rosiglitazone is effective at reducing blood glucose when added to oral monotherapy (metformin or sulphonurea) for patients with type II diabetes who have inadequate blood glucose on these conventional agents alone.

Patients with inadequate blood glucose control on oral monotherapy should first be offered metformin and a sulphonurea unless there are contraindications or tolerability problems. If this is ineffectual and their blood glucose still remains high they should be offered rosiglitazone combination therapy as an alternative to injected insulin.

Answer to question 36

I. Group A beta haemolytic streptococcal infection.

The patient fulfils the Duckett-Jones criteria for acute rheumatic fever, i.e. two major or one major and two minor criteria plus evidence of a recent streptococcal infection.

Duckett-Jones criteria updated 1992
- **Major criteria** include polyarthritis, carditis, erythema marginatum, subcutaneous nodules and chorea.
- **Minor criteria** include fever, arthralgia, raised ESR or CRP and a prolonged PR interval on ECG (if carditis is not a major criteria).
- **Plus evidence of a recent group A streptococcal infection** include isolation of haemolytic streptococci from a throat swab, rising antibody titre (>200 iu/L) or recent scarlet fever.

*Note: the criteria are only to be used for the first episode of rheumatic fever – patients with a previous history need only one major or two minor criteria plus evidence of a streptococcal infection.

The differential diagnosis of rheumatic fever is wide and includes:
- Rubella
- Still's disease
- Hepatitis
- Infective endocarditis
- Sickle cell disease
- Gonococcal arthritis
- Malignancy leukaemia or lymphoma
- Familial Mediterranean fever.

Other notes
- The history and investigations suggest that the patient contracted hepatitis A in Pakistan which had settled before the onset of the current illness (note that there is no significant change in the hepatitis A antibody titres). The raised AST is caused by the rheumatic fever and the elevation is a measure of the severity of the attack.
- Immediate management is bed rest until the arthritis and carditis has settled. All patients should be given penicillin – a singular IM dose of benzathine penicillin or penicillin V bd for 10 days or erythromycin if allergic to penicillin. The dramatic response to salicylate therapy is characteristic of rheumatic fever and patients are routinely given aspirin. Many clinicians use prednisolone in patients with carditis. Cardiac failure will require appropriate treatment.
- Secondary prophylaxis – daily oral or 3-weekly IM penicillin should be continued until 21 years of age or for at least 5 years after the last episode.

2. She is entitled to know his HIV status.

After appropriate counselling it would be ideal if the patient discussed his HIV status with his partner. In the rare exception that he refuses to do this then ultimately there is a legal obligation to inform his partner.

The risk of vertical transmission would be 30% if the pregnant mother was HIV positive.

5. Immune-mediated thombocytopenia.

The most likely cause for this is heparin-induced thrombocytopenia owing to the heparin used in flushes for the indwelling line.

Thrombocytopenia may occur due to decreased platelet production, increased destruction (immunological or other) or sequestration in the spleen.

- Thrombocytopenia may be suggested by a history of excessive bleeding after surgical or dental procedures or recurrent petechiae in the buccal mucosa or at sites of increased intravascular pressure such as the lower extremities. Examination may reveal splenomegaly and lymphadenopathy.
- In acquired thrombocytopenia, platelet size is important because increased bone marrow output is associated with increased platelet size, whereas bone marrow failure is associated with small or normal size platelets.
- Medications can commonly cause thrombocytopenia. This may be due to a myelosuppressive effect – drugs include thiazide diuretics and ethanol. The effect may also be immunological – heparin and quinidine can both cause this.

Heparin can commonly cause a moderate thrombocytopenia ($40–80 \times 10^9$/L) and this typically presents 6–10 days after the administration of heparin, but it can occur earlier if the patient has been exposed to heparin within the last 3 months. Patients often develop venous thrombosis and occasionally arterial thrombosis. The process is mediated by an IgG antibody which recognizes a complex of heparin and platelet factor 4 and initiates platelet aggregation. Unfractionated heparin is more immunogenic than low molecular weight heparin. The diagnosis should always be considered in patients who drop their platelet count after heparin treatment is initiated and in those whose either develop new thrombotic complications or whose established thrombus extends.

Treatment involves stopping heparin and starting an antithrombin agent such as hirudin. Warfarin should not be used in the acute setting as it may lead to warfarin-induced thrombosis.

Common causes of thrombocytopenia
Decreased platelet production
- Aplastic anaemia
- Leukaemia
- Iatrogenic myelosuppression
- Vitamin B_{12}/folate deficiency

Increased platelet destruction
- Non-immune mediated
  - Disseminated intravascular coagulation
  - Heart lung bypass
  - Thrombotic thrombocytopenia
- Immune mediated
  - Drug induced (penicillin, sulfa)
  - Post-transfusion purpura
  - Idiopathic thrombocytopenic purpura*

Hypersplenism (fraction of total platelets in spleen may increase from 30% to 90%)
- Cirrhosis
- Infiltrative diseases

*Idiopathic thrombocytopenic purpura is an acquired condition in which platelet survival is reduced by the presence of platelet-directed autoantibodies.

Autoimmune thrombocytopenia can also occur as part of a systemic autoimmune disease such as systemic lupus erythematosus. It can also be a complication of chronic lymphocytic leukaemia and other lymphoproliferative disorders.

Other notes
- There are a number of congenital causes of thrombocytopenia, these may occur due to infections, toxins or antibodies that a fetus is exposed to in uterine life. The peripheral blood film may show platelets that are small, normal or large in size. Small platelets are uncommon but seen in the Wiskott Aldrich syndrome. Large platelets are common in various other disorders such as the Bernard Soulier syndrome and the May Hegglin anomaly.

3. Lymphangiomyomatosis.

Lymphangiomyomatosis or lymphangioleiomyomatosis (LAM). This is characteristically a disease of premenopausal females that is due to the proliferation of atypical smooth muscle cells in the lung, lymphatics and uterus. Occasional reports document its occurrence in post-menopausal women on hormone replacement therapy. Its aetiology is unknown but a causal role for oestrogens has been proposed. LAM has been described in association with tuberous sclerosis. It presents with dyspnoea due to progressive interstitial lung disease, pneumothorax or chylous pleural effusion. Chylous ascites has been described. One third will have renal angiomyolipomas even in the absence of tuberous sclerosis.

Chest X-ray shows changes as reticular shadowing including Kerley B lines due to dilated lymphatics, small nodules and pleural effusions. Later in the disease, honeycombing and cystic dilation occur, predisposing to pneumothorax.

The pulmonary physiology is similar to that of emphysema (decreased functional vital capacity, increased respiratory volume, and decreased TLCO and KCO).

Diagnosis – the textbook presentation of diffuse cystic change affecting the costophrenic angles in a non-smoking woman of child-bearing age with coexisting renal angiomyolipomas is virtually pathognomonic. However, most would seek tissue confirmation to exclude metastatic sarcoma or atypical Langerhan's cell histiocytosis.

Medroxyprogesterone is used as an anti–oestrogen agent because of the apparent oestrogen dependence of the disease. Pleurodesis may be required. Lung transplantation has been used for advanced disease.

Other notes
- **Langerhan's cell histiocytosis**
  - Langerhan's cell histiocytosis almost exclusively affects smokers between the ages of 20–40 years and is characterized by proliferation of Langerhan's cells. Langerhan's cells are antigen presenting cells and they contain Birbeck bodies seen on EM.
  - The main symptoms are cough, exertional dyspnoea and spontaneous pneumothorax. Wheeze, crackles and clubbing may be present. There may be manifestations of granulomatous infiltration in other organs, particularly in bone and hypothalamus. (A classical presentation, therefore, would be a young male with spontaneous pneumothorax and diabetes insipidus.)
  - Radiologically a reticulonodular infiltrate affecting the middle and

upper zones and sparing the costophrenic angles is typical. Progression leads to cystic change and bullae.

- Lung function tests reveal decreased vital capacity, increased respiratory volume and decreased carbon monoxide transfer. A mixed obstructive and restrictive pattern is often seen.

- The diagnosis may be confirmed by bronchoalveolar lavage with >5% of Langerhan's cells or with lung biopsy.

- The mainstay of treatment is smoking cessation. For patients with progressive disease, steroids and cytotoxics may be used though their effectiveness is variable.

- **Neurofibromatosis** is a recognized cause of basal fibrosis but the patient has none of the clinical features.

- **Alveolar proteinosis** may be primary (M>F) or secondary (e.g. insecticides, silica, aluminium, lymphoma, leukaemia, HIV) and is characterized by accumulation of lipoproteinaceous material in the alveolar space. Clinical features include: dyspnoea, cough, chest pain and haemoptysis, crackles 30%, clubbing 30%. X-rays usually show bilateral infiltrates often in a bat-wing pattern. Bronchoalveolar lavage confirms the clinical diagnosis, yielding milky fluid due to large amounts of PAS positive lipoproteinaceous material.

- **Hermansky Pudlak** syndrome comprises oculocutaneous albinism, abnormal platelet function and interstitial lung disease.

3. Iatrogenic.

This patient has an elevated serum creatinine secondary to trimethoprim. The normal urea makes other explanations more unlikely. Trimethoprim competes with creatinine for excretion by the distal convoluted tubule.

Disproportionate increases in serum urea/creatinine concentration can occur in the following:

Urea > creatinine
Dehydration/ pre-renal failure
Gastrointestinal haemorrhage
Acute on chronic renal failure
Corticosteroids
Tetracyclines
Infection
Post surgery

Creatinine > urea
Liver disease
Trimethroprim/septrin
Cimetidine
Rhabdomyolysis
Dialysis
Race – black
Pregnancy
Vomiting

2. Wenckebach phenomenon.

There is progressive atrioventricular delay (PR interval) until there is one period of complete atrioventricular block, after which the cycle restarts.

Atrioventricular (AV) block occurs when atrial depolarization fails to induce ventricular depolarization due to an anatomical or functional impairment in the conduction system.

There are three degrees of block:
- First degree block describes slowed conduction without missed beats.
- Second degree describes missed beats. There are three varieties:
  1. Type I block in which progressive PR interval prolongation is preceded by a non-conducted P-wave – the Wenkebach phenomenon.
  2. Type II block in which the PR interval remains unchanged prior to the P-wave that suddenly fails to conduct to the ventricles.
  3. When alternate P-waves or every third P-wave is not conducted, i.e 2:1, 3:1 block
- Third degree describes complete AV block.

Type I block most often involves the AV node and is generally benign – it can occur in normal subjects, athletes, the elderly, and in patients with heart disease or who are taking drugs that block the AV node (e.g. digoxin, verapamil, diltiazem, beta blockers). Type II block is almost always below the AV node and can progress to complete heart block. 2:1 and 3:1 block may cause heart failure if the ventricular rate is slow enough. Complete heart block requires a permanent pacemaker insertion.

3. Vitamin C deficiency (scurvy).

The mild thrombocytopenia and minimally prolonged INR are unlikely to account for the signs or for haemorrhage into a single area.

The diagnosis of scurvy requires measurement of plasma and leucocyte ascorbic acid levels.

Deficiency leads to unstable collagen formation resulting in defective perivascular support tissues leading to capillary fragility and poor wound healing. The normal body pool of ascorbic acid is about 1500 mg and 3% of this turns over each day, resulting in a half-life of about 18 days.
  Treatment is with ascorbic acid.

Typical features of ascorbic acid deficiency
- Lassitude, irritability and cognitive impairment
- Perifollicular skin haemorrhage and hyperkeratosis
- Alopecia, coiled fractured corkscrew hair
- Swollen haemorrhagic gums
- Haemorrage into bone giving a periosteal reaction
- Subconjunctival haemorrhage
- Often associated with iron/vitamin B_{12} deficiency, therefore normocytic anaemia.

Other notes
- *Vitamin A deficiency.* Vitamin A is present in the diet as retinal or beta-carotene that is found in leafy vegetables. Deficiency predisposes to gastrointestinal and respiratory tract infections, and night blindness; if it is severe it can result in keratinization of the cornea and corneal ulceration.
- *Vitamin K deficiency.* Vitamin K is found in liver and leafy vegetables and is also synthesized by colonic bacteria. Deficiency is most commonly due to treatment with anticoagulants such as warfarin. The prothrombin time will be raised. Deficiency may also arise in obstructive jaundice.
- *Vitamin E deficiency.* This is a rare complication of steatorrhoea and prolonged parental nutrition. Altered red cell membrane stability can lead to haemolytic anaemia in children; skeletal muscle breakdown can cause a raised CK in adults and children.
- *Niacin deficiency.* This leads to pellagra with diarrhoea, dermatitis, dementia and death.
- *Vitamin B_1 (thiamine) deficiency.* Thiamine, the first B vitamin identified, is referred to as B_1. It is found in yeast, meat, beef, whole grains and nuts. Milled and polished rice contain a small amount. Deficiency initially induces anorexia, irritability, apathy, generalized weakness, pain and parathesia. Prolonged thiamine deficiency causes beriberi, which is classically categorized as 'wet' or 'dry':
  - 'Wet' beriberi presents primarily with cardiovascular symptoms, due

to impaired myocardial energy metabolism and dysautonomia, and can occur after 3 months of a thiamine-deficient diet. Clinical features are an enlarged heart, tachycardia, high-output congestive heart failure, peripheral oedema, and peripheral neuritis.

– 'Dry' beriberi presents with a symmetrical peripheral neuropathy of the motor and sensory systems with diminished reflexes. The neuropathy affects the legs most markedly and patients have difficulty rising from a squatting position.

Alcoholic patients with chronic thiamine deficiency may also have central nervous system manifestations known as Wernicke–Korsakoff encephalopathy.

Answer to question 43

a) 2. Pyschogenic polydipsia.

b) 3. Water deprivation test.

She is normovolaemic, as assessed by physical examination, is hypotonic and hyponatraemic, and is passing very dilute urine. This can only be caused by excess water intake.

- With ADH-dependent water retention the urine osmolality should be high.
- In the case of neurogenic diabetes insipidus the plasma osmolality and sodium are usually normal provided water is freely available; if water is not freely available they are elevated due to increased free water loss.

Summary of expected values for urine osmolality during the water deprivation test (mOsm/kg)		
	Urine osmolality: following water deprivation	Following DDAVP
Normal*	>750	No further rise
Complete cranial diabetes insipidus	<300	Rises by > 50%
Partial cranial diabetes insipidus	300-750 (partial concentration)	Rises by >10%
Nephrogenic diabetes insipidus	<300	No further rise
Psychogenic polydipsia	300-750 (partial concentration)	No further rise (due to medullary washout)
Normal range for plasma osmolality = 278-305 mOsm/kg Normal range for urine osmolality = 60-1500 mOsm/kg		

In **psychogenic polydipsia** the ADH is appropriately low. If there is difficulty in distinguishing between neurogenic diabetes insipidus and psychogenic polydipsia, a water deprivation test should be performed with serial measurement of weight, plasma and urine osmolality and plasma ADH. The plasma osmolality should rise to above 290 mmol/L (to ensure an adequate stimulus for ADH secretion); in the case of true diabetes insipidus the urine osmolality will not increase appropriately. Desmopressin (an analogue of ADH) is then given; a rise in the osmolality of the urine will be seen with neurogenic diabetes insipidus but not with nephrogenic diabetes insipidus. In nephrogenic diabetes insipidus there is end-organ resistance to ADH (ADH levels are typically normal). In some cases of psychogenic polydipsia the results of the water deprivation test may be difficult to interpret. This may be resolved by an infusion of hypertonic saline with serial measurements of plasma and urine osmolalities, along with plasma ADH levels and urine volumes.

1. CH50 total haemolytic complement assay.

The history would be typical of meningococcal meningitis and septicaemia and suggests a previous episode. There is a family history of a similar illness.

These are pointers towards an immune deficiency state. This would be typical presentation of a primary complement deficiency of one of the components of the terminal pathway which often presents with recurrent invasive meningococcal disease.

Terminal pathway complement deficiency is due to an inherited deletion of one of the terminal complement genes (C5–9). This is tested by requesting a CH50 which provides a functional assessment of the classical pathway of complement activation.

The CH50 assesses the integrity of the classical pathway. The patient's sera is added to a standardized suspension of sheep red cells coated with rabbit antibody. Complement is activated via the classical pathway resulting in lysis of sheep red cells; the CH50 is the reciprocal of the serum dilution that lyses 50% of the sheep red blood cells. Homozygous deficiency of a complement component in the classical pathway will result in a CH50 of 0; individual complement levels may then be determined.

Lack of complement-mediated lysis results in inefficient clearance of neisserial infections.

Other notes

- External connections to the cerebrospinal fluid should also always be considered as a cause of recurrent meningitis. These can occur secondary to head injury, erosive sinus disease and after pituitary surgery. Recurrent meningitis can also occur in patients with occult spina bifida.
- Immunoglobulin subclasses would assess whether there was an acquired antibody deficiency such as common variable immunodeficiency (CVID), which typically presents with chronic childhood infections and chronic diarhoea often with giardia lamblia.
- The nitroblue tetrazolium test assesses defective neutrophil function: Chronic granulomatous disease would be an example of this. Patients have chronic suppurative abscesses or granulomas affecting the skin, lung, liver and lymph nodes.
- CD3, -4, -8, -19 lymphocyte markers will quantify total helper and cytotoxic T-cell and B-cell numbers respectively and can assess any deficiencies in their levels.
- Patients with bacterial meningitis may also have other features to support the diagnosis such as pyrexia; neck stiffness; focal neurological deficits; signs of ear or upper respiratory tract infections and papilloedema. The presentation may also be far less typical, patients may complain of severe muscle pain or abdominal pain (due to haemorrhage and impending DIC). A deterioration in their condition may be rapid and fatal.

Answer to question 45

4. Low and high dexamethasone suppression tests.

This patient is likely to have Cushing's disease – an ACTH secreting pituitary micro-adenoma leading to secondary adrenal hyperplasia and hypercortisolaemia.

Clinical symptoms of Cushing's syndrome include weight gain, menstrual irregularity and amenorrhoea, hirsuitism; impotence in the male, depression, muscle weakness and fractures secondary to osteoporosis.

Characteristic signs include: muscle wasting that is often evident as a proximal myopathy, abdominal striae, thin skin, water retention and abnormal fat distrubution (supraclavicular fat pads are well recognized). Hypertension and hyperglycaemia are present in 30% of patients. A hypokalaemic metabolic alkalosis is often present.

Cushing's syndrome may result from:
• Cushing's disease: this describes a pituitary tumour (a microadenoma in 90% of cases) causing raised ACTH levels and secondary adrenal hyperplasia. This is the commonest non-iatrogenic cause and accounts for 80% of cases.

Other causes dependent on ACTH production:
• Ectopic ACTH production: small cell carcinoma of the lung, bronchial adenoma carcinoid tumours, carcinoma of the pancreas, non-teratomatous ovarian tumour
• Iatrogenic ACTH administration
• Very rarely, ectopic corticotrophin releasing hormone.

Causes that are independent of ACTH production:
• Iatrogenic: steroids – likely to be the commonest cause
• Adrenal adenoma and carcinoma
• Carney's syndrome: an autosomal dominant condition comprising mesenchymal tumours (especially atrial myxomas), skin pigmentation, peripheral nerve tumours, endocrine tumours and often adrenocortical dysplasia leading to ACTH independent Cushing's syndrome
• Alcohol: pseudo-Cushing's syndrome.

Investigations
1. **24-urinary free cortisol** measurements are used to demonstrate persistently elevated cortisol levels.
2. **Loss of diurnal variation in plasma cortisol.**
3. **The overnight dexamethasone suppression test**. 1 mg dexamethasone is given at midnight and the cortisol level is checked before and at 8 a.m. If the level suppresses to <50 nmol/L then the diagnosis is unlikely to be Cushing's syndrome. (False positives can occur due to alcohol excess

and drugs which act as inducers of liver enzymes and increase the rate of dexamethasone metabolism. These include phenytoin, phenobarbitol and rifampacin.)

4. **High and low dose dexamethasone suppression tests** can then be used to further investigate suspected cases of Cushing's syndrome. Dexamethasone is a synthetic steroid that in a normal individual would be expected to suppress ACTH secretion from the pituitary. In Cushing's disease (Cushing originally described a pituitary tumour causing raised cortisol levels) the feedback mechanism will be impaired and in adrenal adenomas and ectopic ACTH production the feedback mechanism will be absent.

- **Low dose DXT**: 0.5 mg of dexamethasone is given orally 6-hourly for 48 h. Serum cortisol should suppress below 50% baseline or below 125 nmol/L. Normal individuals and patients with pseudo-Cushing's (obese, depressed or alcoholic) will usually suppress whereas patients with a true Cushing's syndrome will not. This test does not help distinguish between a pituitary adrenal or ectopic cause of raised cortisol levels.

- **High dose DXT**: this can be used to help localize the tumour. Two milligrams of dexamethasone is given 6-hourly for 48 h and again, serum cortisol should be suppressed by 50% or to a level of less then 125 nmol/L. If there is no suppression of cortisol and the plasma ACTH remains high then this would indicate the presence of an ectopic ACTH-secreting tumour. (Most of the pituitary tumours will suppress with the high dose DXT – indicating pituitary disease.)

4. Imaging studies such as CT or MRI can then be used to confirm the presence of a neoplasm but note that adrenal 'incidentalomas' can occur in 1% of normal individuals.

5. Other tests:

- Because the high dose dexamethasone test may not reliably distinguish between Cushings disease and ectopic ACTH syndrome a corticotrophin releasing hormone (CRH) stimulation test is sometimes required. Patients with an ectopic ACTH syndrome typically have no increase in plasma cortisol or ACTH. Patients with pituitary dependent Cushing's disease have an increase in both hormones.

- Inferior petrosal sinus testing for ACTH after stimulation with CRH should show levels that are three times higher then basal levels if there is a pituitary cause.

a) 3. Infective endocarditis.

b) 4. Echocardiogram.

The upper abdominal pain, spleen tenderness and wedge defects are splenic infarcts. The pulsatile left iliac fossa mass is a mycotic aneurysm and this would require further investigation with digital subtraction angiography. The neurological symptoms have resulted from emboli.

Cerebral emboli occur in nearly 20% of cases, typically in the middle cerebral artery territory. The formation of a cerebral mycotic aneurysm is particularly ominous since these have a high chance of rupturing, causing a subarachnoid haemorrhage or intraventricular haemorrhage.

The clinical features of **infective endocarditis** include: fever, evidence of an acute phase response, polyclonal activation of B-cells producing raised rheumatoid factors and a false positive VDRL, petechial haemorrhages, splinter haemorrhages, Osler's nodes (pulp of the finger), Janeway lesions (on the thenar and hypothenar eminence), Roth spots (retinal infarcts), conjunctival haemorrhages, splenomegaly, and clubbing in long-standing cases. Emboli may affect any organ. Renal lesions include both emboli and glomerulonephritis. Effects on the nervous system are due to embolic phenomena. In chronic cases a normochromic normocytic anaemia develops. The WBC may be raised, normal or in severe cases depressed.

In 90% of cases the organism is grown from blood culture; previous antibiotic administration or unusual organisms account for most of the exceptions. Both *Coxiella burnetti* and Mycoplasma may cause endocarditis and can be detected serologically.

The principles of treatment are sterilization of the valve using appropriate antibiotics (usually given for 6 weeks) followed by surgery if the valve is badly damaged. Considerations for early surgery should include infections with organisms such as *Staphylococcus aureus* (most commonly affecting the tricuspid valve in intravenous drug users) or *Streptococcus pneumoniae*, which are characterized by rapid tissue destruction, fungal endocarditis, patients with aortic root infection, and patients with prosthetic valves.

40% of patients will not have previously detected underlying heart disease when they present with endocarditis. Underlying causes may be congential, rheumatic, degenerative or related to mitral valve prolapse. Chronic rheumatic heart disease has now receded as a cause in the west and accounts for less then half of cases. Mitral valve prolapse which is commoner and present in 7–8% of healthy females may account for an increased presentation of endocarditis on this valve and in females. The most common degenerative valve changes are aortic sclerosis or stenosis and mitral annulus calcification. Aortic valve infection occurring in older men is likely to be a result of the increased incidence of aortic sclerosis in this age group.

Congenital heart disease is present in 10% of adults with endocarditis although in children it accounts for the majority.

Summary of some of the commoner congenital cardiac defects	
Defect	Description and clinical features
Atrial septal defect	Ostium secondum defects 90% Ostium primum defects 10%
Patent ductus arteriosis	A left to right shunt is present from proximal to the aortic isthmus to the pulmonary arteries
Ventricular septal defect	Ranging from small defects with no increase in right ventricular pressures to large defects with advanced pulmonary vascular disease and development of shunt reversal (Eisenmenger's syndrome)
Bicuspid aortic valve	Likely to be the most common congenital cardiac lesion
Coarctation of the aorta	Sometimes a feature of Turner's syndrome Gross collateral circulation and associated with hypertension
Tetralagy of Fallot	(i) A large subaortic VSD, (ii) infundibular stenosis leading to, (iii) right ventricular hypertrophy and, (iv) overriding aorta. This leads to (i) cyanosis, (ii) RVH, (iii) single-second sound (aortic) and, (iv) pulmonary ejection systolic murmur

Answer to question 47

a) 5. Cold autoimmune haemolytic anaemia.

The likely diagnosis is idiopathic cold haemaglutinin disease.

b) 1. The direct antiglobulin (Coombs') test is likely to be positive for complement only.

Acrocyanosis, (coldness, purplish discolouration and numbness of fingers, toes, ear lobes and the nose), haemoglobinuria and marked autoaggluttination of red cells, points to a diagnosis of cold autoimmune haemolytic anaemia. The antibody may be monoclonal as in idiopathic cold haemaglutinin disease (CHAD) or polyclonal following infections such as with *Mycoplasma*. Haemolytic anaemia in CHAD is caused by a monoclonal IgM antibody that will agglutinate and lyse (due to the fixation of complement) red cells in the cooler parts of the body – cold antibodies only react with red cells at a temperature below about 32°C and they are most active at about 4°C. In warm autoimmune haemolytic anaemia they are most active at 37°C.

The antibody is usually directed against factor I on the red cells.

Idiopathic cold haemaglutinin disease is a disease of elderly patients. Episodes of painful acrocyanosis and numbness (Raynaud's phenomenon) with a variable degree of intravascular haemolysis are the main features. The blood film made at room temperature shows gross autoagglutination. Autoagglutination would be absent if the blood was prepared at body temperature. The presence of antibody or complement on the surface of the red cell is detected by the direct antiglobulin test, the Coombs' test.

The main treatment is to keep the patient warm and treat the underlying condition. Steroids and splenectomy are not of benefit. Blood transfusion should be avoided if possible; if absolutely necessary, it should be given slowly and via a warming coil.

Other notes
- **Paroxysmal cold haemoglobinuria** is rare and can complicate syphilis and viral infections. The Donath Landsteiner antibody (IgG) is present and binds to red cells in the cold but complement-mediated lysis occurs centrally so acute intravascular haemolysis occurs after cold exposure.
- **Warm autoimmune haemolytic anaemia** is an uncommon disorder that may arise at any age and affects females slightly more than males.
  - It is more common in older age groups because of its association with lymphoid neoplasms.
  - Most patients present with a progressive anaemia or mild jaundice; rarely there is a fulminant illness with intravascular haemolysis. The spleen is usually palpable but rarely attains a large size, except in association with a lymphoma.

- Anaemia and reticulocytosis are common. There may be neutrophilia, often with a left shift, accompanying the massive erythropoietic drive that follows the onset of anaemia. Nucleated red cells may be seen in the peripheral blood. In uncomplicated autoimmune haemolytic anaemia the platelet count is normal or high; again this is a reflection of general marrow drive, but in some patients the platelets are also destroyed by antibody and the haemolysis is accompanied by thrombocytopenia (Evans' syndrome).

- The peripheral blood film may suggest the diagnosis. Spherocytosis occurs in many but not all cases, and the cells may show autoagglutination. This is not always easy to identify in warm autoimmune haemolytic anaemia, in contrast to the massive autoagglutination that occurs on slides made at room temperature from the blood of people with cold haemagglutinin disease.

- Transfusion may be life saving in the acute phase. Corticosteroids are the first measure used to control haemolysis. Prednisolone is effective. Splenectomy is occasionally performed if prednisolone is ineffective.

Secondary causes of autoimmune haemolytic anaemias

Warm	Cold
SLE and other autoimmune disorders	Lymphomas
Lymphomas (particularly CLL and Hodgkin's disease)	Congential and tertiary syphilis
	Infectious mononucleosis
Drugs (methyldopa, mefanamic acid and levodopa)	*Mycoplasma pneumonia**
	Other viral infections
Ovarian teratomas	Idiopathic
Idiopathic	

*An acute intravascular haemolysis associated with the formation of cold agglutinins can occur following *Mycoplasma pneumoniae* infection. The haemolysis appears about 10–14 days after the onset of respiratory symptoms.

a) 5. Theophylline toxicity.

b) 2. Serum potassium.

As she is allergic to penicillin she was given erythromycin by her GP. Erythromycin is an enzyme inhibitor and is recognized to elevate theophylline levels from the therapeutic to the toxic range (theophylline has a narrow therapeutic index). The clinical picture fits well with theophylline toxicity.

The blood gases taken are essentially in the normal ranges. She is not hypoxic and there are no specific risk factors for pulmonary embolism. Hyperventilation would lead to hypocapnoea. Acute severe asthma would be suggested by: PEF 33–50% predicted, inability to complete sentences, respiration rate >25/min, pulse >110/min.

Theophylline toxicity can result in nausea, vomiting, anxiety and agitation, dilated pupils, hyperglycaemia and hypokalaemia.
- It can also lead to convulsions and ventricular and supraventricular arythmias.
- Profound hypokalaemia may develop rapidly.
- Hypokalaemia requires rapid correction and large doses may be required.

The mechanism of action of theophylline is unclear; proposed mechanisms include:

I) Inhibition of phosphodiesterase with increased levels of cAMP relaxing smooth muscle and inhibiting inflammatory cells

II) Competitive antagonism of adenosine at adenosine receptors.

Theophyllines are metabolized in the liver. Their half-life is increased in liver disease, heart failure, viral infections, in the elderly and by enzyme inhibitors, e.g. macrolide antibiotics, cimetidine, ciprofloxacin, fluvoxamine and the oral contraceptive pill. The half-life is decreased in smokers, in chronic alcoholics and in patients on enzyme-inducing drugs such as anticonvulsants and rifampicin.

3. Chronic eosinophilic pneumonia.

The WBC is 10×10^9/L – 40% polymorphs, 15% lymphocytes, leaving 45% which are most likely to be eosinophils. The normal eosinophil count is 0.04 to 0.4×10^9/L.

Leading causes of eosinophilic lung diseases
- Loffler's syndrome
- Acute eosinophilic pneumonia
- Chronic eosinophilic pneumonia
- Allergic bronchopulmonary aspergillosis
- Churg Strauss syndrome
- Bronchocentric granulomatosis
- Idiopathic hypereosinophilic syndrome
- Parasitic infections
- Drugs

Other pulmonary disorders in which peripheral blood eosinophilia (>6% eosinophils), bronchoalveolar lavage eosinophilia (>1%) or tissue eosinophilia occur include: asthma, idiopathic pulmonary fibrosis, hypersensitivity pneumonitis and histiocytosis X.

A significant blood eosinophilia may be seen in lymphoma, chronic myeloid leukaemia and Addison's disease.

Other notes
- *Cryptogenic fibrosing alveolitis* could account for the symptoms but the progression and weight loss had been rapid. The chest X-ray changes would be more likely to show reticulonodular shadowing and it is not associated with a significant eosinophilia of this level.
- *Pulmonary histiocytosis X* occurs almost exclusively in smokers and is characterized by shortness of breath, honeycombing of the lung and pneumothoraces.
- *Lymphangiomyomatosis* occurs in females and the onset will be gradual. The chest X-ray is likely to show reticulonodular shadowing.
- *Loffler's syndrome (simple pulmonary eosinophilia)* is usually a self-limiting illness and weight loss would be unlikely. It typically presents with a cough, sometimes with yellow sputum, or the patient may have no respiratory symptoms.
  - Patients often have a backround history of atopy.
  - There is a modest eosinophilia of between $1–2 \times 10^9$/L. (A differential of more than 20% in a modestly raised WCC would be unusual.)
  - ESR and IgE are usually elevated.
  - The sputum can show an abundance of neutrophils.
  - The pulmonary shadows are transient and are typically peripheral fan-shaped areas of consolidation. Nodules may be present.

- – Underlying parasitic infections can often be found.
- – Drugs such as aspirin, sulphonamides, antimalarials and nitrofurantoin have all been implicated.
- Chronic eosinophilic pneumonia – this tends to run a chronic cause and presents with dyspnoea, fever and weight loss. Associated systemic features are skin and hepatic necrosis and hepatosplenomegaly.
  - – There may be atopic manifestations such as rhinitis, sinusitis and angioedema.
  - – The pulmonary disease is generally extensive.
  - – Radiologically, the shadows may be pneumonic (hence the term eosinophilic pneumonia). The classical textbook description of a photographic negative of pulmonary oedema pattern with extensive dense peripheral infiltrates is seen in approximately 25%.
  - – The pathological presentation is one of macrophages, lymphocytes and polymorphs in the alveolar exudates.

a) 1. Autoimmune chronic active hepatitis.

b) 3. Anti-smooth muscle antibodies and anti-liver-kidney microsome (LKMI) antibodies.

c) 2. Corticosteroids.

This patient has had symptoms of malaise for several months, has several spider naevi and a biochemical hepatitis. The most likely diagnosis in this case is an **autoimmune chronic active hepatitis (CAH)**. Vitiligo, the positive ANA and raised immunoglobulins all suggest an autoimmune aetiology. Corticosteroids form the mainstay of treatment, reduce inflammation in 80–90% of cases and reduce the chance of progression to cirrhosis if it has not already occurred.

CAH is commoner in women than in men and presents in two peaks, between 10 and 25 years of age and between 50 and 65 years of age. In addition to a biochemical hepatitis characterized by a raised alanine aminotransferase level with a normal or only slightly elevated alkaline phosphatase, and the stigmata of chronic liver disease, 50% have other systemic symptoms including fever, arthralgia, vasculitic skin lesions, haemolytic anaemia, thrombocytopenia and leucopenia. A number of patients have other autoimmune diseases such as systemic lupus erythematosus, fibrosing alveolitis, diabetes mellitus, autoimmune thyroid disease, kerato-conjunctivitis sicca and ulcerative colitis. Typically, patients have a positive ANA (titre 1:80 or greater), raised immunoglobulins, primarily IgG, and a high titre of anti-smooth muscle antibodies. Other autoantibodies may be present, in particular to liver-kidney microsomes (LKMI). These appear to be specific for autoimmune chronic active hepatitis.

Liver histology shows inflammation in the portal and periportal areas with 'piecemeal' necrosis. In advanced disease, liver architecture is disrupted and healing with fibrosis eventually leads to a macronodular cirrhosis. Other essential management steps in this patient would also include stopping the contraceptive pill and alcohol, which may be contributing to the liver damage. While immunosuppression with corticosteroids is likely to be used initially; azathioprine may be added as a steroid-sparing agent. In a severe case, with failure of medical treatment, orthotopic liver transplantation should be considered.

Other notes

- The differential diagnosis of chronic hepatitis includes:
  1. Autoimmune hepatitis (often associated with other autoimmune diseases)
  2. Chronic viral hepatitis serological tests available for hepatitis B, hepatitis C and hepatitis D.
  3. Alcohol

4. Drugs, e.g. methyldopa, nitrofurantoin and isoniazid
5. Wilson's disease
6. α_1 anti-trypsin deficiency.
7. Haemachromatosis
8. Sarcoidosis

- Occasionally early primary biliary cirrhosis (PBC) and primary sclerosing cholangitis (PSC) may present with a biochemical hepatitis and be confused with chronic active hepatitis. They are usually differentiated by a predominant elevation in serum alkaline phosphatase and the **anti-mitochondrial antibody** in PBC and the antineutrophil cytoplasmic antibody (ANCA) and changes on cholangiography in PSC. Note, however, that there may be overlap of antibody profiles and also that in 20% of cases the characteristic antibodies may be lacking in CAH.

5. Atrial fibrillation with left bundle branch block.

The ECG demonstrates:
- A broad complex tachycardia with an irregular rate of between 130–200 beats per minute. There are no clear P waves. This would be consistent with atrial fibrillation and left bundle branch block.
- Ventricular tachycardia would be more likely to be characterized by a regular, broad complex tachycardia with concordant QRS complexes pointing downwards in all leads.

Features of left bundle branch block include:
- Wide QRS >120 ms (3 small squares)
- No secondary R wave in lead V1
- No lateral Q waves.

Answer to question 52

3. Thrombotic thrombocytopenia purpura (TTP).

The combination of acute onset neurological abnormalities in association with microangiopathic haemolytic anaemia, thrombocytopenia, and renal failure is highly suggestive of this diagnosis. There may be mild derangement in clotting, but no evidence of disseminated intravascular coagulation.

Thrombotic thrombocytopenic purpura (TTP) is one of the microvascular occlusive disorders. These are characterized by systemic or intrarenal aggregation of platelets, thrombocytopenia and mechanical injury to erythrocytes with high LDH levels. TTP may be familial due to deficiency of a von Willebrand cleaving metalloproteinase (ADAMTS 13) or acquired which may be idiopathic or secondary to systemic lupus erythematosus, ticlopidine, clopidogrel or pregnancy (where IgG Ab to ADAMTS 13 which inhibit its function can be found). Large multiplers of von Willebrand factors cause platelet microvascular thrombi. Typically there is sudden onset of fever, neurological signs, evidence of bleeding and renal failure of varying severity. It is closely related to the haemolytic uraemic syndrome (HUS) of childhood, though neurological involvement is more common. Histologically there is widespread evidence of microvascular hyaline thrombi.

Treatment for familial types involves infusion of platelet-poor fresh frozen plasma to replace ADAMTS 13. Infusions need to be repeated every 3 weeks. For acquired TTP, treatment is plasma exchange to remove the pathological antibodies and the large von Willebrand factors, in addition to the fresh frozen plasma infusion.

Other notes

A microangiopathic haemolytic anaemia describes the mechanical destruction of red blood cells in small blood vessels which arises secondary to changes that include microthrombi, fibrinoid necrosis and malignant cell infiltration. The blood film typically shows microspherocytes and fragmented red cells.

Causes of a microangiopathic haemolytic anaemia include:
- Septicaemia, e.g. meningococcal septicaemia
- Haemolytic uraemic syndrome
- Thrombotic thrombocytopenic purpura
- Malignant hypertension
- Pre-eclampsia
- Renal cortical necrosis
- Acute glomerulonephritis
- Disseminated mucinous carcinomatosis
- Polyarteritis nodosa
- Wegener's granulomatosis
- Systemic lupus erythematosus

TTP and Haemolytic uraemic syndrome:		The Thombotic Microangiopathies	
Expected haematological and biochemical findings:			
Hb	⇓	LDH	⇑
Plts	⇓	+/− deranged renal function	⇑
PT	N	vWF multimers	⇑
APPT	N		
Fibrinogen	N ⇓		
FDP	N		
Schistocytes, and fragmented cells (microangiopathic anaemia)			

Systemic platelet aggregation with greater likelihood of CNS involvement usually termed:	Platelet aggregation confined to the renal circulation more often termed:
TTP ▼	HUS ▼
Microvascular thrombi occur in most organs. These consist of platelet aggregates with little or no fibrin. There is no perivascular inflammation or endothelial damage. Platelet thrombi contain abundant von Willebrand factor multimers that would normally be cleaved, but defects in the required metalloprotease (ADAMTs 13) means that passing platelets adhere to the long multimers and occlusive platelet thrombi are formed.	Exotoxins (released most commonly by *e coli* O157: H7) enter the systemic circulation on the surface of platelets and monocytes. They attach to glomerular capillary endothelial and mesangial cells stimulating the release of TNFα and other interleukins inducing endothelial cells to secrete unusually large von Willebrand multimers. ADAMTS 13 levels are normal. Renal damage is inflicted by monocytes and neutrophils invading the glomeruli in response to the secreted chemokines.
Causes	
• Most often idiopathic • Also recognized with use of Ticlodipine and Clopidogre • Pregnancy and post partum • Others: e.g. SLE	• *e coli* O157: H7 most common in children • *shigella dysentariae* • familial in 5–10% of cases. With a 50% mortality rate. Relapses common. Associated with a complement factor H defect. (It normally protects host cells from damage by the alternative complement pathway.
Treatment	
• In patients who produce functionally defective metalloprotease, episodes of TTP are reversed or prevented by the infusion of platelet poor FFP or cryoprecipitate • Acquired TTP in adults and children requires plasma exchange	• Supportive treatment is required with fluid resuscitation if there is a short lived period of anuria. • Dialysis is more likely to be needed in adults. • Plasma exchange and FFP has had equivocal results. • If there is difficulty distinguishing the disorders plasma exchange should be administered.

Answer to question 53

3. Oat cell carcinoma of the lung.

This patient is hypertensive and, in addition to the raised glucose level, she has a hypokalaemic metabolic alkalosis.

The most likely diagnosis is Cushing's syndrome secondary to ectopic ACTH production and in a 45-year old-smoker the likely ectopic source is an oat cell carcinoma of the lung.

Ectopic ACTH production usually presents with the metabolic features of steroid excess. These are hypertension, diabetes, muscle weakness and a hypokalaemic metabolic alkalosis. In addition, marked pigmentation may occur.

A chest X-ray may reveal the tumour that tend to be proximal, with evidence of invasion of local lymph nodes and local structures with wide dissemination before presentation.

A Plasma ACTH level may confirm the diagnosis of ectopic ACTH production. Typically, very high levels are associated with non-small cell lung cancer (>200 ng/L) and these are accompanied by high plasma cortisol levels (>1000 nmol/L).

1. Commence insulin glargine in place of her evening Insulatard dose.

Insulin glargine (Lantus) is a long-acting insulin analogue which is prepared by modifying the chemical structure of insulin to allow more consistent release of insulin throughout the day, thereby mimicking basal insulin release. The prolonged absorption profile with no peaks allows for a once daily dosing and the possibility of giving bolus injections of short-acting insulin when required, depending on food intake and activity levels. An isophane insulin preparation (such as insulatard) is a suspension of insulin with protamine that has an intermediate duration of action. This may be used for twice daily insulin dosing. Because of a peak in the level of activity at 2–4 h, patients can have particular problems with nocturnal hypoglycaemia.

Biphasic insulin preparations are a combination of a short-acting soluble form of insulin which has a peak action over 2–4 h and a longer-acting preparation which has a peak over 4–12 h and a duration of action over 16–35 h. Commonly used preparations would be Human Mixtard 30/70 (30% soluble (short acting) and 70% isophane (intermediate acting)).

A twice daily regimen in this patient is unlikely to give her the flexibility in dosing that she requires throughout the day. With varying activity levels, she is likely to want to control her level of insulin more closely.

Other notes
- Roseglitazone is not currently licensed for use with insulin. Metformin is often used with insulin in patients with type II diabetes mellitus and has been shown to be effective at reducing insulin requirements and reducing weight gain.

Answer to question 55

a) 2. Wilson's disease.

b) 5. Renal tubular acidosis type II (proximal renal tubular acidosis).

This 17-year-old female has presented with an acute jaundice associated with a normal anion gap metabolic acidosis with appropriate acidification of the urine.

A severe haemolytic anaemia and a fulminant hepatitis is a typical presentation in 10–15% of patients with **Wilson's disease**. It is nearly always fatal without hepatic transplantation. The particular features that help to identify this condition are that it usually causes a rapid deterioration in the patient's clinical state associated with very high bilirubin levels (up to 500 mmol/L) due to both liver failure and an acute haemolysis (a Coombs' negative haemolytic anaemia). The clinical course is characterized by progressive jaundice, ascites, encephalopathy, hypoalbuminaemia and deranged clotting. The liver enzymes may only be moderately elevated or normal.

A proximal renal tubular acidosis is due to proximal bicarbonate wasting but the urine can be appropriately acidified. The urine pH given in this question therefore effectively excludes a distal renal tubular acidosis where there is an inability to acidify the urine to a pH <5.3.

Wilson's disease is an autosomal recessive disorder of copper metabolism where impairment of the normal excretion of copper results in toxic accumulation of the metal in the liver, brain and other organs.

50% of patients will present with hepatic disturbance. They may have an acute hepatitis that is normally self-limiting and can be mistaken for a viral hepatitis or infectious mononucleosis. Parenchymal liver disease may then develop into a clinical picture that is difficult to distinguish from chronic active hepatitis and cirrhosis. The cirrhosis may develop insidiously after a lapse of decades with no prior signs or symptoms of liver disease. A fulminant hepatitis associated with a haemolytic anaemia as described above is also well recognized.

The remainder of patients present with neurological or psychiatric disturbances and are always accompanied by Kayser-Fleischer rings. These are golden deposits of copper in Descemet's membrane.

Neurological manifestations include resting and intention tremors, spasticity, rigidity and chorea. Sensory changes never occur as part of the presentation.

Any form of psychiatric disturbance might occur and this is present in most patients with neurological manifestations.

In a small proportion of patients the first presentation may be primary or secondary amenorrhoea or repeated spontaneous abortions.

The diagnosis is confirmed by the demonstration of either:

- A serum ceruloplasmin level <20 mg/dL *and* Kayser-Fleischer rings or
- A serum ceruloplasmin level <20 mg/dL *and* a concentration of copper in a liver biopsy sample >250 ug/g dry weight
- 24-h copper urine collections will always be raised in Wilson's disease but can also occur in other liver diseases.

Treatment consists of administering a copper-chelating agent such as penicillamine.

In cases where the presentation is of fulminant hepatic failure then a liver transplant will be required.

5. Goodpasture's syndrome (anti-GBM disease).

The differential of a pulmonary–renal syndrome will commonly lie between Wegener's granulomatosis, Goodpasture's syndrome and systemic lupus erythematosus.

The most likely diagnosis in this case is **Goodpasture's syndrome** but the differentiation may be difficult and rely on characteristic serology and/or renal biopsy.

Note that:

- Bacterial pneumonias may also be complicated by a glomerulonephritis.
- Primary renal pathology may have secondary pulmonary effects, e.g. a pulmonary embolism complicating renal vein thrombosis and any cause of acute renal failure may lead to secondary pulmonary oedema.

Goodpasture's syndrome is a combination of rapidly progressive glomerunonephritis and lung haemorrhage, confirmed by the demonstration of autoantibodies to the glomerular basement membrane, which are present in over 90% of patients.

A young male smoker will typically present with cough, breathlessness, and haemoptysis. There is little in the way of generalized systemic disturbance. Renal disease may be missed because it is only evident as proteinuria or microscopic haematuria. The blood pressure is usually normal at presentation. Within a few days or weeks, renal involvement becomes clinically obvious and may progress rapidly to renal failure. The haemoptysis is intermittent and ranges from occasional streaks to massive fatal bleeding.

His chest X-ray will show patchy shadows due to intra-alveolar blood. These shadows may be single or multiple or occur diffusely throughout both lung fields. The shadows resolve over the course of 2 weeks unless there is further bleeding.

He may be hypoxic and have reduced lung volume but gas transfer is increased because inspired carbon monoxide is taken up by blood in the lungs.

Aside from smoking, inhalation of organic hydrocarbons appears to be another provoking factor in exposing the basement membrane to antibody. Immunofluorescence shows a linear deposition of antibody (IgG) along the basement membrane which is usually associated with complement deposition. The glomeruli show focal proliferative and necrotizing glomerulonephritis, usually with crescent formation.

The main treatment is plasma exchange, which must be started early before there is irreversible renal damage and continued until antibasement membrane antibodies are absent, plus corticosteroids and cyclophosphamide. Patients should not smoke and should avoid hydrocarbon exposure. With effective treatment the prognosis is good.

Note: there are three diseases that can cause linear deposition of IgG on the glomerular basement membrane:
   1. *Anti GBM disease (Goodpasture's syndrome)*
   2. *Diabetes mellitus*
   3. *Systemic lupus erythematosus*

Other notes
In a case of **lupus nephritis** the patient (more commonly female) may be hypertensive and would often have evidence of nephrotic range proteinuria. Careful control of hypertension is important because this can become refractory. High dose immunosuppressive therapy is sometimes required.

Legionaire's disease is a pneumonia caused by the organism *Legionella pneumophila*. It is acquired from environmental water sources by the inhalation of water droplets. Typically, the illness starts with acute high fevers, shivers, bad headache and muscle pains. A high fever will be present in 75% of cases. A dry cough and dyspnoea are common. There may be a history of travel or a stay in hospital.
- Non-respiratory features, such as confusion and delirium or diarrhoea occur in more than one-half of patients but respiratory signs are often clinically detectable.
- Focal neurological signs, particularly of a cerebellar type, are well described but meningitis does not occur.
- Proteinuria, microscopic haematuria, and casts are found in 20–30%.
- Shock, rhabdomyolysis, endotoxaemia, and disseminated intravascular coagulation can lead to acute renal failure.
- Renal biopsy typically shows an acute interstitial nephritis or acute tubular necrosis.
- The WCC is moderately raised, often with a lymphopenia. Hyponatraemia, hypoalbuminaemia, and abnormality of liver function tests are present in 50%. Gram stain of sputum stain typically shows few pus cells and no predominant pathogen; initial blood and sputum cultures are negative unless dual infection is present.
- Radiographic shadowing is usually homogeneous and commonly confined to one of the lower lobes on presentation. Characteristically, radiographic deterioration occurs with spread of shadows both within the same lung and to the opposite side. A small pleural effusion can occur in one-quarter of cases. The most important pulmonary complication is acute respiratory failure requiring assisted ventilation, which occurs in up to 20% of patients.
- The diagnosis may be made on the detection of urinary antigen (sensitivity

70% for Legionella serogroup 1), serology may be useful, but peak levels can take 2 to 4 weeks leading to a delay in the diagnosis and sputum culture.
- Preferred antimicrobials– clarithromycin or ciprofloxacin; alternatively doxycycline.

Differentiation of various pneumonias on clinical grounds is therefore not specific. The features in the following box are those most closely associated with each pathogen:

Pathogen	Features
Streptococcus pneumoniae	Increasing age, comorbidity, acute onset, high fever and pleuritic chest pain
Bacteraemic Streptococcus pneumoniae	Female sex, excess alcohol, diabetes mellitus, chronic obstructive airways disease, dry cough
Legionella pneumophila	Younger patients, smokers, absence of comorbidity, diarrhoea, neurological symptoms, more severe infection, evidence of multisystem involvement (e.g. abnormal liver function tests, elevated creatinine kinase)
Mycoplasma pneumoniae	Younger patients, prior antibiotics, less multisystem involvement
Chlamydia pneumoniae	Longer duration of symptoms before hospital admission, headache
Coxiella burnetti	Male sex, dry cough, fever

Wegener's granulomatosis is a necrotizing granulomatous vasculitis which involves both the upper and lower respiratory tracts. Typically this is accompanied by a small-vessel vasculitis affecting the kidney, and to a variable extent other organs.
- Circulating autoantibodies to neutrophil cytoplasmic antigens, usually to proteinase 3 (c-ANCA), can be found in 90% of untreated patients at presentation.
- Patients may develop a bloody, foul-smelling nasal discharge, paranasal sinus pain, nasal ulceration and septal perforation, which may lead to the characteristic saddle-shaped deformity of the nose. They may also develop a chronic suppurative otitis media, due to eustachian tube blockage, a chronic non-productive cough, dyspnoea, pleurisy, and haemoptysis, which all reflect vasculitic injury and/or development of granulomata in the airways or lung parenchyma.
- Chest X-rays characteristically show pulmonary nodules which may cavitate, or patchy shadows due to intra-alveolar haemorrhage.
- Asymptomatic proteinuria and haematuria is the first indicator of renal involvement.
- A focal necrotizing glomerular capillaritis with crescent formation is the histological hallmark of a rapidly progressive nephritis and is characteristic of Wegener's granulomatosis, which may be indicated by red cell casts in the urine.

Other features:

- Conjunctivitis, uveitis, and scleritis may all occur
- In a patient with proptosis, (due to a retro-orbital granuloma) combined with lung or renal disease, think of Wegener's granulomatosis
- An arthritis can develop but joint deformity is not a feature
- A variety of lesions can be found in the skin. These may vary from nailfold infarcts and purpuric rashes to isolated ulcers, vesicles and papules
- Mononeuritis multiplex is the commonest neurological lesion.

Buerger's disease (thromboangitiis obliterans) is a thrombotic disorder of medium-sized vessel vasculitis that occurs almost exclusively in smokers and that leads to limb ischaemia.

Answer to question 57

4. Serum insulin-like growth factor-1 (IGF-1).

Her history suggests that she may have **acromegaly**: she has diabetes, is hypertensive, and has enlargement of her hands and a proximal myopathy.

Acromegaly is due to hypersecretion of growth hormone from a pituitary tumour. It usually presents between the ages of 30–50 years and the onset may be insidious. Most features are due to growth of the soft tissues: coarse oily skin, large tongue, prominent supraorbital ridge, 'spade-like hands', deepening voice, arthralgia, progressive heart failure and sleep apnoea. There may also be features of a pituitary tumour. Sweating and headache are also common. Complications include: diabetes mellitus, hypertension, cardiomyopathy. The definitive test is the OGTT **with** GH measurement; normally GH levels would be suppressed but in acromegaly there is no suppression or an increase in the GH level. Serum IGF-1 is a reliable screen for acromegaly and an elevated level would support the clinical diagnosis. Growth hormone secretion is pulsatile and therefore random levels are of limited use. The action of growth hormone on tissue is mediated in an endocrine manner via hepatically-derived IGF-1. Its levels are therefore elevated in patients with acromegaly although there is no stong correlation between the clinical feature of acromegaly and the serum concentrations of IGF-1.

Other notes
- Pituitary function tests may reveal hypopituitarism.
- Visual field analysis may reveal optic nerve compression and a typical bitemporal hemianopia.
- The treatment of choice is transphenoidal surgery. Prior to the introduction of surgery, dopamine agonists proved the mainstay of treatment but response rates are not good in comparison with the use of dopamine agonist in patients with prolactinomas. The somatostatin analogue octreotide is now regularly used to treat patients and this is administered subcutaneously.

The **carpal tunnel syndrome** should be suspected with a history of tingling confined to the radial digits. This is caused by elevated pressure in the carpal tunnel, causing ischaemia of the median nerve. It is associated with a variety of conditions. These include:
- Pregnancy
- Inflammatory arthritis
- Colles' fracture
- Amyloidosis
- Hypothyroidism
- Diabetes mellitus
- Acromegaly
- Cushing's syndrome.

There are a number of commonly used clinical tests to try and detect a carpal tunnel syndrome. These include:

1. Loss of two point discrimination in the median nerve distribution and associated thenar wasting although these typically occur late in the disease.

2. In Phalen's test the patient reports whether flexion of the wrist for 60 s elicits pain or paraethesiae in the median nerve distribution.

3. Tinel's sign is where tapping over the volar surface of the wrist causes radiating paraethesia.

   Due to the variable sensitivity and specificity of these tests, electrodiagnostic studies are the most reliable in confirming a diagnosis and excluding other neuropathies.

The differential diagnosis of discomfort in the hand includes entrapment of the nerves, (such as carpal tunnel syndrome, entrapment of the ulnar nerve and cervical radiculopathy), tendon disorders and arthropathies.

a) 4. Rhabdomyolysis.

b) 2. Status epilepticus.

Rhabdomyolysis secondary to status epilepticus and a period of unconsciousness is the most likely diagnosis.

Rhabdomyolysis may also occur with sepsis, trauma, after prolonged exertion and following burns and electrocution. Biochemically it is characterized by a massively disproportionate rise in serum creatinine from muscle damage compared with blood urea, hyperkalaemia, increased muscle enzymes (AST and CPK), hypocalcaemia as a consequence of calcium binding to damaged muscle, and hyperuricaemia. Myoglobin is detected in the urine and if in high enough concentration will turn the urine 'coca cola' red-brown. Myoglobinuria gives a false positive dipstick result for blood but can be distinguished from haemoglobinuria by the ammonium sulphate test, which gives a coloured precipitate with haemoglobinuria and a coloured supernatant with myoglobinuria. Treatment is principally supportive, although alkalinization of the urine may ameliorate tubular damage and the development of acute tubular necrosis; the renal lesion will resolve spontaneously but a period of dialysis may be necessary. Non-symptomatic hypocalcaemia should not be treated, as the calcium will deposit uselessly in the muscle.

2. Scl–70 antibody.

The most likely antibody to be positive in this patient is Scl - 70 (anti topsiomerase-1). The clinical presentation is typical of diffuse cutaneous systemic sclerosis.

Systemic sclerosis is a heterogenous rheumatic disease where there is fibosis of the skin and internal organs with a microvasculopathy.

The presentation of disease varies from localized plaques of skin involvement (such as linear scleroderma and morphoea) to generalized 'systemic sclerosis' affecting multiple organ systems. The generalized variety is also subdivided into limited cutaneous and diffuse cutaneous systemic sclerosis depending on the degree of skin disease.

There may also be overlap with other disorders such as systemic lupus erythematosus, polmyositis and arthritis. Cases can also present with little or no skin involvement and these are termed 'systemic sclerosis sine scleroderma'.

Limited cutaneous systemic sclerosis typically presents with a long history of Raynaud's phenomenon, which can be severe and associated with digital ulceration. Other manifestations include oesophageal dysmotility and gastrooesophageal reflux and patients typically have subcutaneous telangectasia and subcutaneous calcinois. **Skin involvement is distal** and does not progress above the elbows or knees although the face is involved. Patients may have features consistent with the CREST syndrome (Calcinosis, Raynaud's phenomenon, oEsophageal dysmotility and Telangectasia) but this term is used less commonly because it ignores other systemic manisfestations of the disease. Up to 70% of patients will be positive for anti-centromere antibodies.

In diffuse cutaneous systemic sclerosis there is skin involvement **proximal** to the elbows and knees symptoms of Raynaud's phenomenon and oesophageal involvement are present and internal organs can be severely affected. Lung involvement and hypertensive renal crises are common. Many patients will be positive for anti-topsoimerase antibodies are present in up to 40%.

Main serum autoantibodies found in scleroderma and their most significant clinical associations		
Antigen	Most significant association	Main organ involvement
Scl-70 Topsoimerase I	Diffuse	Lung fibrosis
Centromere	Limited	Pulmonary hypertension Severe gut disease
RNA polymerase I, II and III	Diffuse	Renal and skin disease
U3RNP	Overlap	Pulmonary hypertension and muscle
U1RNP	Limited, overlap and Afrocarribeans	Pulmonary hypertension and small bowel
PM - Scl	Overlap	Mixed, muscle

a) 4. **Ventricular septal defect with a right-to-left shunt.**

b) 4. **Pulmonary regurgitation**

There is pulmonary hypertension (normal 25), elevated right ventricular pressure (normal 25) with a right-to-left shunt (left ventricular oxygen saturations less than aorta, indicating venous mix at ventricular level). The most common cause is an **Eisenmenger ventricular septal defect.**

The Eisenmenger complex occurs because the high pulmonary blood flows due to a left-to-right shunt lead to progressive increases in pulmonary pressures leading to pulmonary hypertension and subsequent shunt reversal. According to Eisenmenger's original description, this is also associated with tricuspid regurgitation and the development of a pan-systolic murmur secondary to this (rather then the large VSD where there is not enough turbulent flow to cause a murmur).

The low pulmonary artery diastolic pressure suggests pulmonary regurgitation. This often occurs as a result of prolonged pulmonary hypertension. There is no systolic gradient.

Note: closure of the ventricular septal defect at this stage would lead to rapid death from right ventricular failure. With pulmonary vascular resistance of this magnitude the right ventricle is protected from fatal dilation and failure by the 'offloading' effect of the tricuspid incompetence and the systolic right-to-left shunt.

Answer to question 61

a) 2. X-linked recessive.

According to the family tree, males are affected and unaffected females are able to transmit the trait. Therefore the likely mode of transmission is X-linked recessive.

An abnormal gene carried on one of the X chromosomes in a female will be passed on to half of her daughters, who would be heterozygous like herself, and to half of her sons, who would manifest the disease because they have no compensating X chromosome. An affected male would produce only heterozygous daughters, but cannot pass the gene on to his sons, who only receive his Y chromosome.

b) Patient A) 1. Not affected.

The risk to patient A and his children is zero as he will receive a Y chromosome from his affected father. We can assume that the chance that a new mutation would give rise to the same condition can be ignored.

b) Patient B) 3. 1:4.

In the case of patient B, his great-grandfather was affected, implying that his grandmother was a carrier and therefore the probability that his mother was a carrier is 1:2; his risk is therefore 1:4.

b) Patient C) 3. 1:4.

The mother of patient C has an affected brother, therefore the probability that she is a carrier is 1:2; the chance that her daughter will also be a carrier is 1:4.

Other notes
The most common X-linked recessive conditions are haemophilia A and B, Duchenne and Becker's muscular dystrophy and glucose-6-dehydrogenase deficiency. Other conditions that are X-linked recessive are nephrogenic diabetes insipidus, Hunter's syndrome, Lesch–Nyhan syndrome, colour blindness and Fabry's disease, and the fragile X syndrome.

4. Chronic renal failure.

Chronic renal failure explains the mild hyperkalaemia and acidosis, the hypocalcaemia and the normochromic normocytic anaemia. Most patients with chronic renal failure will have a low T4 and T3 but a normal TSH and TRH response. The T4 tends to normalize once effective renal replacement therapy is introduced.

Causes of galactorrhoea include:
1. Pregnancy
2. Antidopaminergic drugs – e.g. phenothiazines, butyrophenones, metoclopramide, methyldopa
3. Oestrogens
4. Hypothalamic/pituitary lesions
5. Hypothyroidism
6. Chronic renal failure
7. Ectopic prolactin secretion, e.g. bronchogenic carcinoma, hypernephroma.

a) 4. MRI lumbar spine.

b) 5. Lumbar canal stenosis.

There are a number of mechanisms that may lead to stenosis of the lumbar canal. These include osteoarthritis with hypertrophy of the facet joints, disc prolapse, surgery, spondylolisthesis, Paget's disease, neoplasia and infection. Any of these conditions may be superimposed on a congenitally narrow spinal canal.

Typically the symptoms develop slowly and may be very vague. Back pain, as such, is not a feature. The neurological symptoms often do not fit into any clear root or peripheral nerve distribution. In chronic cases there may be quadriceps wasting. The A–P diameter of the lumbar spinal canal is narrowed during extension, which appears to interfere with the blood supply to the cord; by stooping forward the A–P diameter is increased, therefore rapidly relieving the symptoms.

Normal plain radiographs of the spine do not exclude the diagnosis. Intermittent claudication may easily be distinguished from this syndrome by Doppler examination of the pulses before and after exercise.

Surgery is often very effective in relieving symptoms and increasing exercise tolerance.

a) 4. Phenytoin toxicity.

She has developed phenytoin toxicity, presenting with a cerebellar syndrome, mild megaloblastic anaemia and osteomalacia. The recent fit might be paradoxical, i.e. related to high phenytoin levels. Rifampicin is an enzyme inducer and when coprescribed with phenytoin, it usually lowers serum phenytoin levels. Her attending physician had anticipated this and asked her to increase her daily dose by 30%; unfortunately she had misunderstood the instructions and was taking three times her previous daily dose. Note: isoniazid is an enzyme inhibitor and to some extent will negate the effect of rifampicin

b) 4. Phenytoin levels.

A raised phenytoin level would confirm the diagnosis.

The principal side-effects of phenytoin include:
1. Central nervous system: cerebellar signs, typically ataxia, tremor, nystagmus and dysarthria; sedation; mood swings; peripheral neuropathy; increased fits
2. Haematological: folate deficiency leading to a megaloblastic anaemia; aplastic anaemia; lymphadenopathy
3. Endocrine: increased metabolism of vitamin D which may lead to osteomalacia; reduced ADH levels, worsening of diabetes mellitus
4. Skin: acne; coarsening of facial features; gum hypertrophy; Dupuytren's contractures
5. Hepatitis
6. Drug-induced lupus
7. Drug fever
8. Fetal abnormalities: microcephaly, congenital heart disease, cleft palate and hare lip
9. Phenytoin is an enzyme inducer and will increase the metabolism of drugs such as the oral contraceptive pill.

Answer to question 65

a) 3. Right Holmes-Adie pupil.

b) 4. Diminished reflexes.

c) 4. Idiopathic.

The Holmes-Adie pupil is a benign condition, which occurs mostly in women and is unilateral in 80% of cases. The affected pupil is moderately dilated. The pupil reacts sluggishly to light and sometimes not at all. It slowly reacts to accommodation and may eventually constrict more than the normal pupil. It is often associated with absent or diminished ankle and knee reflexes.

The Argyll-Robertson pupil occurs in neurosyphilis. The pupil is constricted and is unreactive to light, but reacts to accommodation. This can also occur in diabetes.

Optic neuritis or glioma presents with diminished visual acuity and an afferent pupillary defect. Light shone in the affected eye does not cause direct or consensual pupillary constriction.

Other notes

Causes of a dilated pupil
- Third nerve palsy
- Mydriatic eye drops
- Holmes-Adie pupil
- Iridectomy
- Brain stem death

Causes of a constricted pupil
- Old age
- Pilocarpine eye drops
- Horner's syndrome
- Argyll-Robertson pupil
- Pontine lesions
- Narcotics

a) 4. Familial hypocalciuric hypercalcaemia (FHH).

b) 4. No treatment required.

Elevated serum calcium (sometimes >3.5 mmol/L), normal or slightly low phosphate, and borderline hypermagnesaemia (0.95-1.10 mmol/L) are typical of **familial hypocalciuric Hypercalcaemia (FHH)**. Three-quarters of patients have a 24-h urinary Ca excretion of less than 2.5 mmoL, which is clearly inappropriate in the context of serum *hyper*calcaemia. A patient with primary hyperparathyroidism would be expected to have an elevated urinary calcium excretion. A serum PTH should be measured. This is normal or mildly elevated in FHH. Vitamin D levels are usually normal. Evaluation of the ratio between urinary calcium clearance and creatinine clearance can help to distinguish between FHH and primary hyperparathyroidism. In the former >80% of subjects have a CaCl/CrCl ratio of <0.01. The majority of patients with primary hyperparathyroidism have values that are higher.

It has been estimated that up to 10% of patients who undergo 'successful' parathyroid surgery have FHH, and patients should be warned about inappropriate surgery. A low calcium diet is not indicated, and management is generally conservative.

Many patients with FHH have specific inactivating mutations in the calcium-sensing receptor gene (often encoding defects in the extracellular part of the receptor). The mutation makes the receptor less sensitive to calcium. In the parathyroid glands this means that a higher than normal serum calcium is required to reduce PTH release. Calcium resorption within the kidney at a given blood calcium level is also enhanced. Some patients have other mutations and genetic analysis is complex. If a kindred with FHH is identified, referral to a specialist centre is indicated.

Answer to question 67

a) 2. Alveolar haemorrhage.

b) 3. Microscopic polyangiitis.

Microscopic polyangiitis is a small vessel necrotizing vasculitis without granuloma formation.

There is a marked elevation in the KCO suggesting **alveolar haemorrhage,** which can occur in the absence of frank haemoptysis.

Goodpasture's syndrome, Wegener's granulomatosis, microscopic polyarteritis and systemic lupus erythematosus can all present with pulmonary haemorrhage.

There are a number of other conditions that may result in raised TLCO and KCO: these are tests of gas exchange. The total gas exchange will be reduced in any case where the alveolar area is diminished with either loss of lung volume such as in lung resection; or when there is loss of alveoli such as in emphysema; or where the capillaries are diseased such as in vasculitic conditions.

The KCO represents the transfer coefficient and is the uptake of CO per litre of lung volume; it therefore corrects for any real or effective reduction in lung volume.

The TCLO and KCO can increase, usually as a result of an increase in red cells to the lungs due to greater blood flow, as a result of haemorrhage, or due to polycythaemia.

Patients with extra pulmonary restriction effectively have an increased density of pulmonary capillaries in relation to the restricted lung volume, so elevating the TLCO and KCO.

Causes of an increased TLCO and KCO		
	↑TLCO	↑ KCO
Asthma	+/−	+ In some cases*
Pneumonectomy	−	+
Extrapulmonary restriction	+	+
Pleural disease	−	+
Rib cage deformity	+	+
Respiratory muscle weakness	+	+
Left-to-right shunts	+	+
Polycythemia	+	+
Lung Haemorrhage	+	+

*In asthma the KCO is normal or increased. The possible reduction in TLCO is because of a misdistribution of ventilation due to airway narrowing.

a) 3. Leptospirosis.

b) 2. IV benzylpenicillin.

Leptospirosis should be considered in any patient presenting with myalgia, fever and conjunctival suffusion, particularly if there is a history of water or animal contact.

In addition this patient has thrombocytopenia, renal failure and jaundice (Weil's disease). It is unusual for the other causes of jaundice such as viral hepatitis, infectious mononucleosis, malaria, legionnaire's disease or brucellosis to present with this triad but these diagnoses should be actively excluded. Leptospirosis, a spirochaetal disease (caused by the *Leptospira interrogans* complex) is carried by rodents and usually passed to humans by contact with rat urine or blood, typically occurring in those exposed to rat excreta in the context of their occupation.

The clinical presentation varies from the classic picture of Weil's disease with multi-organ involvement, to a mild anicteric febrile illness with or without meningism. Clinical features include sore throat, fever, lymphadenopathy, headache, photophobia, conjunctival injection, uveitis, abdominal wall pain (may mimick an acute abdomen), diarrhoea, hepatomegaly, splenomegaly and profound myalgia. Renal involvement occurs in approximately 50% of cases and varies from mild proteinuria to dialysis-dependent renal failure. Jaundice occurs in 10% of cases and is typically due to an elevated conjugated fraction. Pulmonary involvement is common, though the severity varies from a dry cough to marked pulmonary infiltration with respiratory failure and lung haemorrhage.

The diagnosis of leptospirosis is usually made on serology. Isolation of leptospires from the blood or cerebrospinal fluid may be made in the first 10 days of the illness by culture of blood or cerebrospinal fluid but special media is needed. Urine cultures become positive from the 2nd week. A peripheral blood polymorphonuclear leucocytosis is usual.

The cerebrospinal fluid findings: a normal sugar, slightly elevated protein with a pleocytosis.

Intravenous benzylpenicillin is the treatment of choice for patients with severe disease or who are vomiting. Supportive treatment with attention to fluid balance is essential. Dialysis may be necessary. Overall the prognosis is good; poor prognostic factors include severe jaundice, disseminated intravascular coagulation, renal failure and respiratory failure. Patients with mild disease can be treated with oral doxycycline.

Answer to question 69

1. Wolff-Parkinson-White syndrome type A.

There is an obvious delta wave which is positive in lead V1.

The Wolff Parkinson White (WPW) syndrome is a pre-excitation disorder caused by an accessory-conducting pathway directly connecting the atria to the ventricles and bypassing the AV node. In the WPW syndrome AV conduction through the bypass tract (the bundle of Kent) results in earlier activation (pre-excitation) of the ventricles. The PR interval is therefore short (<0.12 s) due to rapid AV conduction through the accessory pathway. The QRS complex consists of fusion between early ventricular activation caused by pre-excitation and later ventricular activation through the usual AV nodal transmission. The slurred upstroke is termed the delta wave.

Two types of QRS patterns were originally identified in patients with the WPW syndrome:
- Type A, due to a left-sided bypass tract, in which there is a tall R wave in leads V1–V3 (i.e. a positive or upward delta wave)
- Type B, due to a right-sided bypass tract in which there are QS complexes in leads V1–V3 (i.e. a negative or downward delta wave).

2. It is most likely that he is poorly compliant with treatment.

Multidrug 'highly active antiretroviral therapy' (HAART) reduces the incidence of opportunistic infections and slows the progression from HIV to AIDS and from AIDS to death.

A combination of agents produces more complete viral suppression and this helps to limit the emergence of drug resistance. Common combinations for triple combination therapies are:

- Triple nucleoside reverse transcriptase inhibitor (NRTI) regimens
- Non-nucleoside reverse transcriptase inhibitor (NNRTI) regimens (which can consist of 2NRTI and 1NNRTI)
- Protease inhibitor based regimens.

Effective antiretroviral therapy should suppress the viral load below detection and CD4 counts should rise. This usually leads to preservation or restoration of immune function.

HAART can suppress HIV type I viraemia to undetectable levels for 3 years or more; during this treatment period low level viral replication continues. Deciding when to commence treatment remains controversial. Generally treatment is deferred if the CD4 count is >350 cells/µL irrespective of the viral load and treatment should definitely be commenced with a CD4 count of <200 cells/µL.

Patients should be monitored by serial measurement of the viral load. If the viral load remains above 10 000 copies/mL, adherence to therapy, drug levels and viral resistance should be assessed. FBC, biochemical profile, lipid levels, lactate and blood glucose should also be carefully monitored.

Lipodystrophy, dyslipidaemia and insulin resistance may complicate protease-inhibitor-containing antiretroviral therapy. This has also led to concerns about long-term cardiovascular complications. The 'lipodystrophy syndrome' describes changes in body fat distribution – typical clinical findings include central obesity, a 'buffalo hump' and characteristic facial thinning. This may also occur with NRTI therapy and is occasionally present in treatment-naïve patients.

Other common side effects of antiretroviral therapy include:

- Lactic acidosis
- Hepatic derangement
- Hyperglycaemia and diabetes mellitus
- Rash
- Neuropsychiatric disturbances

3. Cytomegalovirus infection

The onset of **cytomegalovirus (CMV)** disease is usually 30–90 days after transplantation. CMV produces its most severe manifestations in immunosuppressed patients, especially patients with AIDS, post-solid organ transplantation and in bone marrow recipients.

Clinical features include interstitial pneumonia, bone marrow suppression or graft failure.

Patients can also develop fevers with or without arthralgias, myalgias and oesophagitis. CMV ulcerations can also occur in the upper and lower gastrointestinal tract and diarrhoea can also be a common presentation. In bone marrow transplant recipients it can be difficult to distinguish diarrhoea due to CMV from graft versus host disease.

The risk of CMV disease is much higher in a sero-negative patient receiving a graft from a sero-positive donor and most centres will try to match sero-negative donors with sero-negative recipients.

Treatment options include ganciclovir and foscarnet.

Other considerations in immunocompromised patients

The diagnosis of pneumonia in recipients requires consideration of the fact that patients have undergone treatment with multiple chemotherapeutic agents and sometimes radiation. The differential should include: bacterial pneumonia – CMV pneumonitis, pneumonia of other viral or fungal aetiology, parasitic pneumonia, diffuse alveolar haemorrhage and chemical or radiation associated pneumonitis. Tuberculosis is uncommon in patients without a backround predisposition.

Differential diagnosis of chest infiltrates in Immunocompromised patients		
Infiltrate	Infectious	Non-infectious
Localized	Common bacterial pathogens, *Legionella*, mycobacteria	Local haemorrhage or embolism
Nodular	Fungi: *Aspergillus* or *Mucormycosis Nocardia*	Recurrent neoplasia
Diffuse	*Viruses, CMV, Chlamydia, Pneumocystis cariini, Toxoplasma gondii, Mycobacteria*	Congestive cardiac failure, radiation pneumonitis, drug-induced lung injury, diffuse alveolar haemorrhage

a) 3. Systemic lupus erythematosus.

- Remember that there are three diseases in which linear IgG deposition may be reported on the glomerular basement membrane: (i) diabetes mellitus, (ii) systemic lupus erythematosus (SLE) and iii) anti-GBM disease (Goodpasture's syndrome).
- Goodpasture's syndrome is unlikely with this degree of hypertension and nephrotic range proteinuria, and is more common in male patients.
- Diabetes mellitus is made unlikely with a normal glycosylated Hb level.
- Refractory hypertension is common in lupus nephritis and an important pitfall in its diagnosis is the apparently innocuous urinary sediment underlying an aggressive nephritis.

b) 3. Membranous nephritis.

Sub-endothelial and intramembranous deposits typical of diffuse membranous glomerulonephritis.

Lupus nephritis is now classified according to the histological features:
Class I – normal on light microscopy
Class II – mesangial disease with hypercellularity
Class III – focal segmental glomerulonephritis
(<50% of glomeruli involved)
Class IV – diffuse proliferative glomerulonephritis
(>50% of glomeruli involved)
Class V – diffuse membranous nephropathy.
Class VI – advanced sclerosing glomerulonephritis

The management of membranous glomerulonephritis in the context of SLE is controversial. Patients with active SLE and impaired renal function should be treated aggressively with corticosteroids and cyclophosphamide or mycophenolate. Attention should be given to aggressive control of blood pressure and hyperlipidaemia.

Answer to question 73

a) 2. Insulinoma.

b) 3. CT scan of the pancreas.

The patient is hypoglycaemic with an elevated insulin and C-peptide – diagnostic of endogenous insulin secretion.

With a blood glucose of 2.4 mmol/L, plasma insulin level should be <3 mU/L. In this case the important differential diagnosis is exogenous insulin administration. The latter can be excluded by the measurement of plasma-immunoreactive C-peptide which will be low in the case of exogenous insulin and high with an endogenous source.

An **insulinoma** is the commonest cause of excess insulin secretion and non-diabetic fasting-induced hypoglycaemia. These are tumours of B cells and can occur in any part of the pancreas. The majority are benign and slow growing. 10% are malignant. Median age of presentation is the 5th decade. Patients typically present with drowsiness on waking and eating something relieves this. Other modes of presentation include fits, dizziness, diplopia and paraesthesia. Patients may become obese as their calorie consumption increases in an attempt to avoid symptoms.

A 72-h fast and serial measurement of glucose, insulin and C-peptide levels may be of use in patients with a suggestive history. Seventy to eighty percent of patients with an insulinoma will develop hypoglycaemia during the first 24 h and 98% by 48 h.

Spontaneous hypoglycaemia can be divided into two groups: (a) fasting hypoglycaemia and (b) post-prandial or reactive hypoglycaemia.

A) **Fasting hypoglycaemia** – symptoms occur at night, in the early morning or after a fast. This group can be subdivided into:
● Excess insulin production or self-administration (no ketosis):
  – Insulinoma, excess exogenous insulin, retroperitoneal fibrosarcoma*, mesothelioma*
● Non-insulin-induced causes (ketonaemia is a feature) e.g:
  – Liver failure, Addison's disease, hypopituitarism, ethanol, aspirin, propranolol, septicaemia, malaria, autoimmune hypoglycaemia – insulin receptor autoantibodies, end-stage renal disease.

*Retroperitoneal fibrosarcoma and mesothelioma induce hypoglycaemia by induction of insulin-like growth factors.

B) **Post-prandial or reactive hypoglycaemia** – symptoms occur 2–4 h after eating. Causes include:
  – Post gastrectomy, hereditary fructose intolerance.

3. Bartter's syndrome.

The patient is normotensive and investigations show a hypochloraemic hypokalaemic alkalosis together with high urine potassium loss.

Bartter originally described a syndrome of hyperplasia of the juxtaglomerular complex associated with hyperaldosteronism and a hypokalaemic alkalosis.

Molecular genetic techniques have now classified Bartter's syndrome into three types, all of which are autosomal recessive and caused by mutations of Na/K+ pumps in the thick ascending limb of the renal tubule.

Many patients who were previously thought to have had Bartter's syndrome actually had Gittleman's syndrome. This is due to a defect in the Na/Cl-transporter in the distal convoluted tubule (giving a similar biochemical picture to that caused by thiazide diuretics). Gittleman's syndrome also has an autosomal recessive pattern of inheritance. It usually presents in childhood with weakness, vomiting, polyuria, nocturnal enuresis, growth retardation and low IQ.

The overall diagnosis of an inherited potassium wasting disease depends on the demonstration of renal potassium loss in the presence of a hypokalaemic metabolic alkalosis, and sometimes elevated aldosterone secretion and increased plasma renin activity, in a normotensive individual. Abnormal potassium loss in the urine is suggested by the finding of more than 20 mmol of potassium in the urine per 24 h with plasma potassium of less than 3 mmol/L.

Treatment consists of potassium supplementation with or without an aldosterone antagonist. Non-steroidal antiinflammatory agents that interfere with tubular prostaglandin production have been shown to correct the hypokalaemic alkalosis and hyper-reninism. Some patients have hypomagnesaemia and require magnesium supplements.

Differential diagnosis of a metabolic hypokalaemic alkalosis

Adrenal tumours
- The blood pressure would usually be high

Elevated ACTH levels
- Cushings syndrome

Diuretic abuse
- Can be detected on urinary assays

Villous adenoma, laxative abuse

- Both associated with diarrhoea and the urine potassium excretion would be low

Pyloric stenosis – (gastric outlet obstruction)

- HCl is lost from the stomach leading to an alkalosis. (There is increased HCl synthesis and increased bicarbonate secretion into the extracellular fluid)
- Hypokalaemia results from gut loss, alkalosis (potassium shift into cells) and increased urinary loss
- (The reduced chloride concentration limits Na resorption. Na is then exchanged for K+ in the distal tubule)

Bartter's syndrome/Gittleman's syndrome

- The cardinal features are a profound hypokalaemic alkalosis with urinary potassium and chloride wasting in a normotensive individual. There can also be secondary hyperaldosteronism and resistance to the pressor effects of angiotensin II and hypertrophy and hyperplasia of the juxtaglomerular apparatus of the kidneys.

Other causes: liquorice ingestion, hypomagnesaemia

5. Prolonged QT interval.

The ECG shows prolonged QT intervals (about 520 ms).
A collapse during exercise raises the possibility of aortic stenosis, hypertrophic cardiomyopathy or an exercise-induced arrhythmia. This ECG does not show the pattern of left ventricular hypertrophy, making aortic stenosis unlikely.

Any unexplained syncopal episode without evidence of an underlying cause requires further investigation. The long QT syndrome may present with a syncopal episode as a result of short-lived ventricular arrhythmia and, in particular, the development of torsades de pointes. Such patients may not present until they are exposed to medications that prolong the QT interval or to exercise. Erythromycin can prolong the QT interval.

Long QT syndrome
The QT interval is the total time from the onset of ventricular depolarization to the completion of repolarization (the start of the Q wave to the end of the T wave). The length of the QT interval varies with the heart rate and its corrected value may be calculated:

$$QTc = QT/ \text{ Square of RR interval (normal 350–430 ms)}$$

In most circumstances, however, an uncorrected QT length of >450 ms is likely to be pathological.
The main importance of QT prolongation is the associated risk of developing ventricular tachycardias and in particular torsade de pointes; this is an atypical ventricular tachycardia characterized by a continuously varying QRS axis that may generate into ventricular fibrillation. The combination of a long QT interval during sinus rhythm with intermittent torsade de pointes is termed the long QT syndrome.
Prolongation of the QT interval is found in the following:
- Congenital ion channel disorders all show an autosomal dominant mode of inheritance. The most common are: Jervell-Lange-Nielson syndrome and the Romano-Ward syndrome.
- Acquired causes are commonly drug related and may be caused by: quinidine, procainamide, sotolol, amiodarone, tricyclic antidepressants, phenothiazines, erythromycin and fluconazole.
- Other disorders include:
  - Electrolyte disturbances: hypokalaemia, hypomagnesaemia and hypocalcaemia
  - Endocrine abnormalities: hypothyroidism
  - Bradyarythmias: complete atrioventricular block and sick sinus syndrome
  - Other medical conditions: anorexia nervosa, hypothermia, liquid protein diets, ischaemic heart disease and mitral valve disease.

a) 3. Benign intracranial hypertension.

This is the syndrome of an elevation in cerebrospinal fluid pressure in the absence of ventricular dilation or an intracerebral mass.

- Benign intracranial hypertension is predominantly a disease of obese females.
- The aetiology is unknown, though associations with pregnancy, drugs (e.g. tetracyclines, nalidixic acid), dural sinus thrombosis and previous head injury states have been noted.
- Headache is the most common symptom and is universally present. Symptoms of papilloedema are transient visual obscurations and patients may also have horizontal diplopia due to VIth cranial nerve palsies.
- Neurological signs are usually confined to swollen optic discs. A partial VI nerve palsy secondary to raised intracranial pressure (false localizing sign) is found in 30%.
- Visual field analysis is of paramount importance in both the initial assessment and follow-up of patients with benign intracranial hypertension. Typically, patients have blind spot enlargement, constriction of the visual fields and scotoma caused by optic nerve damage.
- A CT scan of the brain will exclude a space-occupying lesion and will show normal or small-sized ventricles.
- Lumbar puncture will then demonstrate an elevated cerebrospinal fluid pressure.
- Dural sinus thrombosis should be excluded by MRI venography. In large centres MRI is the initial investigation of choice and will exclude space-occupying lesions and venous sinus thrombosis.
- The commonest complication is visual loss due to optic atrophy. Permanent visual loss occurs in up to 50% of cases and may be severe in 10%.

b) 4. Diuretics.

Diuretics form the mainstay of pharmacological treatment. Therapeutic lumbar punctures may be performed and high-dose corticosteroids have been used initially to reduce intracranial pressure effectively. Surgery is not usually required, though ventriculoperitoneal shunting of cerebrospinal fluid may be needed if visual loss is progressive and the response to steroids is slow. Optic nerve sheath fenestration has been performed on occasions to decompress the optic nerves.

Most cases undergo clinical remission either spontaneously or in response to treatment, although cerebrospinal fluid pressure may remain high.

4. Renal amyloidosis.

The patient has developed AA amyloidosis as a consequence of chronic osteomyelitis.

Amyloidosis is a well-recognized cause of chronic renal failure and normal-sized kidneys. It is a disorder of protein metabolism characterized by extracellular deposition of abnormal protein fibrils. Accumulation causes disruption to the structure and function of organs and tissues.

Amyloid AA amyloidosis associated with chronic disease

Amyloid AA amyloidosis occurs in association with chronic inflammatory disorders and chronic local or systemic microbial infections, e.g. chronic osteomyelitis and malignant neoplasms. It causes complications in 10% of patients with rheumatoid arthritis.

The most common presentation is with non-selective proteinuria due to glomerular deposition – it may cause nephrotic syndrome before terminating in end-stage renal failure.

Patients may also present with organomegaly, most commonly hepatosplenomegaly. Involvement of the gatrointestinal tract is common in such cases but is not usually the presenting feature.

AL amyloidosis associated with immunocyte dyscrasia

- Multiple myeloma, malignant lymphomas, macroglobulinaemia and benign monoclonal gammopathy may be complicated by immunoglobulin light chain (AL) amyloidosis.
- The majority of patients with AL amyloid have light chains in the urine.
- Patients with myeloma associated with AL amyloid have a significantly worse prognosis.
- The typical patient is a Caucasion male over 50 years. He is likely to present with cardiac dysfunction (90% of cases). There will be evidence of a restrictive cardiomyopathy; arrythmias are therefore common. Gut involvement can cause malabsorption. Macroglossia is virtually pathogonomic. He may have a painful sensory neuropathy.
- The histological diagnosis of amyloidosis is made by observing the green birefringence of deposits stained with Congo red and viewed with polarized light.
- Serum amyloid P scanning is also highly sensitive and can be sufficient to confirm the diagnosis.

Other notes

- Hepatitis C is strongly associated with mixed cryoglobulinaemia and can cause a membranoproliferative glomerulonephritis in patients who will invariably present with purpuric skin lesions, which can become confluent and necrose. Other frequent symptoms are fever, arthralgia and Raynaud's phenomenon.
- The diagnosis would be confirmed with evidence of cryoprecipitation. There is also a specific complement pattern. A high rheumatoid factor titre and a very low C4 with a normal/low C3 would be characteristic.

1. Ultrasound abdomen.

- PKD type 1 accounts for 85% of cases of adult polycystic kidney disease. **Renal ultrasound** reveals bilateral renal cysts in 100% of affected individuals aged 30 years or more. In this variant of PKD, ultrasound will miss cysts in the vast majority of affected children.
- In PKD type 2, the second largest group of patients with adult polycystic kidney disease, renal cysts appear much later, therefore ultrasound as well as CT scan may miss cases, even at the age of 30 years.
- Although genetic testing is possible for the PKD 1 locus it is not practical for non-PKD 1.

Adult polycystic kidney disease (PKD) is an autosomal dominant condition. The predominant morphological abnormalities are the development of cortical and medullary cysts on the kidneys; hepatic cysts and intracranial aneurysms can also develop.

- The most common extrarenal manifestation is colonic diverticulae. Twenty five percent of patients also have mitral valve prolapse. The most serious association is with intracranial aneurysms which may rupture giving rise to either subarachnoid or intracranial haemorrhages.
- The disease may present at any age but characteristically produces symptoms in the 3rd or 4th decade. Patients may develop chronic flank pain from the mass effect of large kidneys. Acute pain can develop as a result of superadded infection, urinary tract obstruction by clot or stone or sudden haemorrhage into a cyst.
- PKD accounts for about 10% of end-stage renal disease. Hypertension is common and patients then have a much more rapid progression to renal failure. About 50% of patients develop end-stage renal failure by the age of 60 years.
- A family history of sudden death or subarachnoid haemorrhage may be the presenting feature of PKD. Screening of all patients with APKD for intracranial aneurysma is controversial but with the increasing availability of non-invasive techniques such as magnetic resonance angiography, patients with a positive family history of subarachnid haemorrhage should certainly be screened.
- Autosomal dominant polycystic kidney disease-1 (ADPKD-1) is due to a defect on the short arm of chromosome 16.
- Autosomal dominant polycystic kidney disease-2 (ADPKD-2) maps to chromosome 4.
- The genes code for a polycystin complex which is thought to regulate cell matrix interactions.

a) 4. Acute pancreatitis.

b) 2. Serum amylase.

The low albumin, low corrected calcium, hypoxia and high blood glucose all point to the diagnosis, which may be confirmed by measurement of serum amylase levels; a level >1000 Somogyi units is said to be diagnostic.

Thiazide diuretics are a recognized cause of acute pancreatitis. Other drugs that might precipitate an acute attack include steroids, azathioprine and the contraceptive pill. In the UK the majority of cases of acute pancreatitis are idiopathic. The commonest-known precipitating cause is gallstones. Other precipitating factors include: alcohol; viral infections, particularly mumps; trauma which may be local, e.g. following ERCP or following general surgery or as a result of carcinoma of the pancreas; hyperparathyroidism; hypertriglyceridaemia and hypothermia.

a) 2. Patent ductus arteriosus (PDA).

b) 4. Angiographic embolization.

A PDA can be large or small. A large PDA can lead to secondary pulmonary hypertension and shunt reversal. If it is small, then it can be asymptomatic. There is a step up in oxygen saturations between RV and PA, indicating a shunt at this level.

Angiographic embolization is used for adults. NSAIDs are used in premature infants.

a) 2. Paroxysmal nocturnal haemoglobinuria (PNH).

b) 4. Ham's test (acid lysis test).

This measures the sensitivity of red blood cells to complement lysis. The patient's red cells are incubated with acidified (which activates complement) fresh autologous serum. More recently the recognition that cell surface regulatory proteins are deficient has led to confirmation of the diagnosis by flow cytometry using antibodies to GPI (glycosyl-phosphatidyl-(Inosityl) linked proteins such as CD55 and CD59.

A right ultrasound Doppler or venogram of the patient's leg veins would be required to confirm the presence of the right deep vein thrombosis.

The occurrence of a thrombotic episode in a patient with pancytopenia is highly suggestive of paroxysmal nocturnal haemoglobinuria. This diagnosis is also suggested by the history of dark urine passed early in the morning, and intermittent abdominal pain.

Paroxysmal nocturnal haemoglobinuria (PNH) is an acquired clonal disorder that is characterized by a chronic haemolytic anaemia, thrombotic episodes and often a pancytopenia.

It occurs due to a defect in the formation of a phosphatidylinosital anchor on the cell surface and the subsequent loss of membrane proteins, including inhibiters of complement (decay accelerating factor (DAF) and membrane inhibitor of reactive lysis (MIRL)). Red cells are therefore unusually sensitive to the complement cascade and intravascular complement-mediated lysis.

PNH can sometimes develop during the recovery phase of an acute aplastic anaemia.

The typical history is of intermittent nocturnal haemolysis leading to dark urine. The haemolysis may be profound and life threatening.

The mechanism behind an increased incidence of thrombosis is not clear but may reflect the susceptibility of platelets to complement activation. Other important sites for thrombosis include hepatic vein obstruction, producing the Budd-Chiari syndrome, and cerebral thrombosis. Intermittent episodes of abdominal pain are thought to result from small thromboses affecting portal blood vessels.

The severity of the symptoms varies; some patients require regular blood transfusions. Corticosteroids and androgens have been used in an effort to control the degree of haemolysis, and iron supplements are necessary as a result of the considerable haemosiderinuria. Anticoagulation is necessary for thrombotic episodes. In some patients the condition is self-limiting as the abnormal clone disappears. Allogeneic bone marrow transplantation has been successfully performed in patients with severe disease.

Other notes
- **Systemic lupus erythematosus** in association with antiphospholipid antibodies is a well-recognized cause of arterial and venous thrombosis and a pancytopenia.

Answer to question 82

a) 3. Multiple sclerosis.

The current presentation would be consistent with acute optic neuritis. The previous symptoms are suggestive of isolated neurological episodes. Resolved cerebral or spinal cord pathology would explain the previous episode of foot dragging, and brainstem involvement often produces symptoms which may be confused with vestibular labarynthitis. An initial relapsing/remitting course is typical of demyelinating disease.

The development of optic neuritis is not synonymous with multiple sclerosis (MS), however between 50–80% of patients may go on to develop classical MS. Periventricular white matter abnormalities are found in 60% of patients with optic neuritis; the presence of these and a positive cerebrospinal fluid analysis for oligoclonal bands during an episode are particularly strong risk factors for progression to MS.

b) 1. Reduced colour vision.

Given the clinical context, the history of left eye pain (present in 90%) and blurred vision is indicative of a left optic neuritis. There will therefore be diminished acuity and decreased colour vision in the affected eye, particularly centrally. Optic disc swelling is present in 35% of patients. Examination of both eyes may reveal nystagmus and/or an internuclear ophthalmoplegia.

c) 3. Magnetic resonance imaging of the head and spinal cord.

This would be the most useful investigation and is likely to show periventricular and spinal cord high signal lesions consistent with areas of demyelination.
- Other investigations would include cerebrospinal fluid analysis for oligoclonal bands.
- Demyelination can also be detected by using visual, auditory, somatosensory and central motor electrophysiological studies.
- The treatment of MS can be divided into:
  1. Treatment for acute relapses such as optic neuritis – usually corticosteriods. (corticosteroids lead to more rapid visual recovery but at the end of a 6-month period the visual acuity is no better then without treatment)
  2. Symptomatic treatment (spasticity, bladder dysfunction, fatigue)
  3. Immunomodulatory treatment – Beta-interferon has been used with variable benefit on relapse rate and reduced disability progression.

Other notes
- Optic neuritis describes optic nerve inflammation due to an idiopathic process or due to an underlying demyelinating or infectious aetiology. In most cases the optic disc is normal on opthalmoscopy and the term retrobulbar neuritis is used. If the optic disc is swollen then this may be termed papillitis or anterior optic neuritis.

3. Congestive cardiac failure.

The biochemical picture of low serum sodium, low potassium, high bicarbonate and elevated urea is explained by the secondary hyperaldosteronism that complicates severe congestive cardiac failure. Note that although serum sodium levels are low, total body serum sodium levels are high. The grossly oedematous intestinal mucosa leads to a protein-losing enteropathy and this explains the hypoalbuminaemia. Oral drugs are often ineffective in such cases due to decreased absorption, and drugs need to be given intravenously.

3. Primary Biliary Cirrhosis.

The patient presents with a cholestatic hepatitis, hepatosplenomegaly, and an upper gastrointestinal haemorrhage. In addition she has an elevated serum IgM and her calcium is at the lower limit of normal (corrected Ca 2.0 mmol/L for an albumin of 40) with a low serum phosphate suggesting early osteomalacia. Patients with primary biliary cirrhosis tend to have few stigmata of chronic liver disease compared with alcoholic liver disease or chronic active hepatitis.

Further investigations should include upper gastrointestinal endoscopy to distinguish between a peptic ulcer and bleeding varices (an enlarged spleen suggests portal hypertension), anti-mitochondrial antibodies and a liver biopsy to confirm the diagnosis of primary biliary cirrhosis, and vitamin D/PTH level to evaluate the low calcium.

Primary biliary cirrhosis chiefly affects females between 30 and 60 years of age, and is second only to alcohol as a cause of chronic liver disease in such patients. It may present with deranged liver function tests, pruritus, jaundice, abdominal pain, anorexia, weight loss, diarrhoea, osteopenia (and bone pain), and evidence of liver failure or upper gastrointestinal bleeding (increased incidence of peptic ulceration). Xanthelasma are common and in chronic cases patients may be clubbed. The natural history is variable: asymptomatic patients may never develop significant disease. Symptomatic patients, e.g. those who present with pruritus, generally progress to cirrhosis with portal hypertension over 7–10 years. Why some patients have a non-progressive form of primary biliary cirrhosis is unknown.

The alkaline phosphatase and γ-GT are raised in >99% of patients; the alanine transaminase and aspartate aminotransferase are usually normal. Bilirubin rises late and suggests a poor prognosis. An elevated IgM is found in 80%, IgG in 40% and IgA only rarely.

Anti-mitochondrial antibodies are positive in >90% of cases; the titre does not have prognostic significance; only four antimitochondrial antibodies, M2, M4, M8 (associated with a worse prognosis) and anti-M9 are associated with primary biliary cirrhosis. Anti-smooth muscle antibody positivity or a weakly positive anti-nuclear factor are also common. A strongly positive anti-smooth muscle antibody or ANA is associated with a phenotype showing features of both chronic active lupoid hepatitis and primary biliary cirrhosis.

Histologically the disease is patchy. The earliest lesion is T-cell mediated focal damage to the interlobular bile ducts with associated granuloma formation, followed by bile duct obliteration/proliferation, fibrosis and finally cirrhosis.

Pruritus may be treated with cholestyramine, antihistamines, or if these fail, rifampicin or UV-radiation; rarely, haemoperfusion is necessary. Liver transplantation is now firmly established as the treatment for end-stage primary biliary cirrhosis. D-penicillamine may produce an improvement in the short term but it is not sustained. Prednisolone improves the biochemical picture but increases osteopenia, hence it should only be used with caution. Osteomalacia may be prevented with calcium and vitamin D supplements. Occasionally the other fat-soluble vitamins are reduced and cause symptoms: vitamin K (bruising), vitamin E (neuropathy), and vitamin A (night blindness). High cholesterol levels will require dietary modification.

Answer to question 85

a) 4. Pseudohypoparathyroidism.

b) 5. Infusion of PTH with measurement of urinary phosphate and cyclic AMP.

The biochemical findings of hypocalcaemia with an elevated phosphate and a normal alkaline phosphatase (normal for a 7-year-old boy) are typical. The differential diagnosis includes primary hypoparathyroidism and pseudohypoparathyroidism (the typical phenotype of pseudohypoparathyroidism includes an oval face and short 4th and 5th metacarpal bones).

The diagnosis of pseudohypoparathyroidism may be confirmed by the Ellsworth Howard test – a PTH infusion fails to increase urine phosphate and cyclic AMP, in contrast to primary hypoparathyroidism where both are elevated.

Note: it would be clinically appropriate to first measure the serum PTH levels which will be absent in primary hypoparathyroidism, and present in pseudohypoparathyroidism, where the abnormality is a failure to respond to PTH hence the abnormal PTH infusion test.

a) 4. Subarachnoid haemorrhage.

Subarachnoid haemorrhage (SAH) is most likely. The patient gives a history of a headache of acute onset – a severe and explosive headache occurring without warning (thunderclap) is typical of SAH.

Focal neurological symptoms can occur when there is haemorrhage into the appropriate cortical areas.

Symptoms and signs of meningeal irritation, if present, are more likely to occur after a few hours as inflammatory blood products migrate to the infratentoral dural lining.

b) 2. CT scan of head.

This is the first line of investigation and is sensitive in 95% of cases to the presence of SAH when taken within 24 h of the onset of headache; thereafter the sensitivity reduces. CT scans may demonstrate the underlying source of the bleed and any space-occupying lesions requiring drainage. Lumbar puncture is necessary in cases of suspected SAH when CT is normal.

SAH can be detected by the presence of xanthochromia between 6 and 12 h after haemorrhage. To ensure that xanthochromia is detected after SAH, lumbar puncture should be deferred until 12 h after the onset of headache. In cases of late presentation after SAH, all patients have xanthochromia up to 2 weeks after haemorrhage, 70% after 3 weeks and 40% after 4 weeks. (Note: 48 h after a SAH there may be a reactive cerebrospinal fluid leucocytosis and low sugar.)

Digital subtraction angiography (DSA) remains the gold standard for investigating the underlying vascular abnormality. CT and MRI angiography are non-invasive tests and are being used with more frequency but they have not fully replaced DSA in most centres.

c) 4. Intracranial aneurysm.

The commonest sites are the anterior communicating artery 30%, middle cerebral artery 25% and posterior communicating 25%; 15% have multiple aneurysms; 5% bleed from arteriovenous malformations.

d) 2. Nimodipine.

Nimodipine is a possible neuroprotective agent and cerebral calcium antagonist. It is at present the only pharmacological agent that has shown any clinical benefit by reducing the frequency of cerebral ischaemia. A 4-hourly oral dose of 60 mg is given. If the patient is comatosed, intravenous nimodipine can be administered, providing hypotension has been corrected. Surgery may be required in the acute resuscitation process if there is evidence of raised intracranial pressure requiring the insertion of an external ventricular drain.

Referral to a neurosurgical centre for further investigation and management is always indicated. Re-bleeds commonly occur at around 1 week, and may be fatal. If technically possible, surgical clipping or coiling of an aneurysm is performed. If no lesion is identified at angiography, management is conservative.

Answer to question 87

a) 2. Alpha-1-antitrypsin deficiency.

b) 4. Alpha-1-antitrypsin electrophoresis.

The lung function tests display an obstructive defect with reduced gas transfer and hyperinflated lungs, manifest by the preserved TLC. The chest X-ray is indicative of basal emphysema. Although the liver may be displaced due to hyperinflated lung fields the palpable spleen indicates that the patient is more likely to have hepatosplenomegaly.

The combination of lung and liver pathology in a patient of this age narrows the differential to either cystic fibrosis or alpha-1-antitrypsin deficiency.

The emphysematous findings are more in keeping with alpha-1-antitrypsin deficiency which classically produces changes maximal at the lung bases: Cystic fibrosis is more likely to present with findings in the lungs consistent with bronchiectasis.

Alpha-1-antitrypsin deficiency is an autosomal recessive disorder. The absence or decreased levels of this protease inhibitor lead to progressive alveolar and liver damage.

- There are a number of different alleles leading to a variable expression. M is the normal allele. Z and S are the most frequently encountered abnormal alleles. Mutations are inherited in a Mendelian fashion – the normal phenotype is therefore PiMM and a heterozygote PiMZ, etc. Each of the deficiency genes results in a decrease in the concentration of alpha-1-antitrypsin. A level of alpha-1-antitrypsin greater then 40% is required for normality. The S variant forms >60% of PiMM and the Z variant 15%. The common heterozygous states MZ (60%) and MS(80%) and SS(60%) do not result in a clinical effect. The SZ 37.5% and ZZ 15% are therefore predisposed to emphysema with the ZZ genotypes being more severely affected.
- The primary role of antitrypsin is to inhibit neutrophil elastase. Without this patients are predisposed to panacinar emphysema.
- The usual presentation is progressive shortness of breath at the age of 50 years in a non-smoker and 30 years in a smoker who has the PiZZ genotype.
- Only the PiZZ phenotype is prone to cirrhosis and all PiZZ individuals have progressive hepatic damage. 80% of this phenotype will have shown evidence of liver damage as a child.
- Alpha-1-antitrypsin deficiency is also associated with an increased incidence of bronchiectasis, glomerulonephritis and a panniculitis.

Other notes

- **Gaucher's disease** is a lysosomal storage disorder which is due to a catalytic deficiency of glucocerebrosidase. It presents with pancytopenia, with bleeding due to thrombocytopenia; splenic enlargement and areas of infarction in the bone lead to painful episodes and avascular necrosis. Rarely pulmonary infiltrates including reticulonodular opacities and a restrictive lung defect can occur.

- **Kartagener's syndrome** is an autosomal recessive condition that leads to repeated sinus and respiratory tract infections, which progress to lung suppuration and bronchiectasis; it is also associated with male infertility and situs inversus.

3. Normal variant.

The abnormalities on the ECG recording are raised ST segments in leads I, II, VL, V3–V6 with high take off ST segments in leads V3–V5. There is also T wave inversion in lead III.

Other causes of ST segment elevation and their associated clinical features

Acute pericarditis
- Diffuse saddle shaped ST segment elevation
- Possible reciprocal ST segment depression in AVR
- Possible PR segment depression

Left bundle branch block
- ST segment deviation discordant from the direction of the QRS

Left ventricular hypertrophy
- Voltage criteria for LVH

Hyperkalaemia
- Widened QRS complexes
- Tall tented T waves

Pulmonary embolism
- Changes simulating myocardial infarction in both the inferior and anteroseptal leads

Acute myocardial infarction
- ST segment elevation with reciprocal changes between AVL and lead III

Prinzmetal's angina
- Transient ST segment elevation

Brugada syndrome*
- Downsloping ST segment elevation in leads V1 and V2 with a right bundle RSR pattern in V1 and V2

*A syndrome linked to mutations in the cardiac sodium channel gene that is associated with cardiac arrest and sudden death.

Note: Cocaine use is a well recognised cause of coronary artery spasm

a) 2. Familial hypophosphataemic rickets.

b) 3. X-linked dominant.

c) 2. A 50%, B nil.

In B, the mother has two normal X chromosomes.

Tubular resorption of phosphate is defective, leading to low plasma phosphate levels. Phosphate deficiency is the primary cause of the osteomalacia, which is characterized in these patients by a raised ALP but usually a normal or minimally-reduced plasma calcium concentration. Since the calcium is relatively normal there is rarely evidence of hyperparathyroidism. The diagnosis may be confirmed by showing an inappropriate phosphaturia. Treatment is large doses of phosphate and if necessary a small dose of vitamin D.

4. Myelodysplasia.

The presence of a macrocytic anaemia, neutropenia and thrombocytopenia suggests a diagnosis of **myelodysplasia**. This diagnosis is supported by the presence of Pelger cells and circulating blasts. The Pelger-Huet anomaly describes neutrophils with reduced nucleus segmentation (single or bilobed). Pelger-Huet cells may rarely be inherited.

It is now recognized that there is a 7 to 10-fold increase in the incidence of acute myeloid leukaemia after intensive chemotherapy for Hodgkin's disease. These leukaemias are usually preceded by myelodysplasia. The risk of developing leukaemia is greatest 5 years after treatment but remains high for up to 8 years after the last course of chemotherapy. An increased risk of acute myeloid leukaemia also occurs in other diseases such as myeloma, polycythaemia rubra vera and carcinoma of the ovary and breast where alkylating agents are used. Such secondary leukaemias are often associated with particular karyotypes such as partial or complete loss of chromosome 5, 7 or Y or trisomy 8. The long arm of chromosome 5 encodes a series of haemopoietic growth factors and differentiation antigens, and its deletion raises fascinating questions concerning the mechanism of secondary leukaemia.

Immunosuppression with non-alkylating agents, as in recipients of renal or cardiac transplantation, is associated with an increased risk of non-Hodgkin's lymphoma.

Answer to question 91

a) 2. Dilated cardiomyopathy.

b) 2. Alcohol abuse.

In relation to alcohol abuse, note the high MCV and low platelet Count. This patient has cardiomegaly with a poor ejection fraction and secondary mitral regurgitation due to dilation.

Dilated cardiomyopathy may be caused by:
- X-linked inheritance (rare)
- Post viral
- Autoimmune
- Toxins, e.g. alcohol
- Drugs: cytotoxics and tricyclic antidepressants
- Puerperal heart failure
- Thyrotoxicosis (rarely)
- Prolonged hypocalcaemia
- Haemochromatosis

a) 4. Right lobe of cerebellum.

The neurological features are consistent with cerebellar disease. A unilateral cerebellar lesion will produce classic cerebellar signs on the same side as the lesion.

The most important physical sign of cerebellar disease is ataxia. This is defined as uncoordinated or inaccurate movement that is not due to weakness, spasticity or intrusion of involuntary movements. Tremor is also an important feature of cerebellar disease – it is a non-rhythmic tremor that appears on action and is therefore called an intention tremor. Nystagmus also commonly occurs with cerebellar disease. In the case of disease of the cerebellar hemisphere, nystagmus will be maximal towards the side of the lesion.

b) 4. Von Hippel–Lindau disease.

The combination of polycythaemia and cerebellar signs suggests a diagnosis of **Von Hippel–Lindau disease**. This is inherited in an autosomal dominant fashion. Haemangioblastomas develop throughout the central nervous system but show a predilection for the cerebellum. Von Hippel–Lindau disease is one of the recognized causes of ectopic erythropoietin production. Other recognized features include: (i) cysts affecting the kidney, liver and pancreas, (ii) renal cell carcinoma, and (iii) phaeochromocytoma.

Other notes
- **Friederich's ataxia** is an inherited condition (AR or sex-linked) causing spinocerebellar and cortical tract degeneration. There is also peripheral nerve degeneration. Patients typically present in their teens with gait ataxia. Other features include pes cavus, scoliosis and optic atrophy. Death occurs due to cardiomyopathy.
- **Refsum's disease** is characterized by polyneuritis, night blindness due to retinitis pigmentosa, sensorineural deafness, cerebellar ataxia and a high cerebrospinal fluid protein.
- **Medulloblastoma** is a mid-line cerebellar tumour that arises from the inferior part of the vermis, causing truncal ataxia and sudden falls.
- **Von Recklinghausen's disease** is characterized by an overgrowth of Schwann cells and fibroblasts, causing neurofibromas, nodules over perphieral nerves, café-au-lait spots, axillary freckling, optic gliomas, acoustic neuromas and honeycomb lung.

Answer to question 93

a) 3. Ventricular septal defect.

There is intracardiac shunting from right to left. The most marked effect of a shunt on saturation is in the chamber beyond that receiving the shunted blood; in this case it is the femoral artery, suggesting a ventricular septal defect.

b) 2. Pulmonary stenosis.

There is a marked peak-to-peak systolic gradient across the pulmonary valve, indicating stenosis.

c) 5. Overriding aorta.

There is demonstrable ventricular septal defect, pulmonary stenosis and right ventricular hypertrophy; the most likely diagnosis is Fallot's tetralogy.

Dizzy spells may represent:
1. Increased right-to-left shunting with reduced peripheral vascular resistance (exercise) and therefore increasing systemic desaturation
2. Recurrent paradoxical emboli which are common due to polycythaemia and the right-to-left shunt
3. Recurrent paroxysmal arrhythmias as a result of atrial distension.

a) 3. Cystic fibrosis

b) 3. A sweat test,   4. Immunoglobulins.

He has evidence of malabsorption, chronic respiratory symptoms, a dilated right colon, and is small for his age. The most likely diagnosis is cystic fibrosis.

Investigations should include a chloride sweat test and this will confirm the diagnosis in 98% of cases – the characteristic defect is that secretions contain too little water relative to the protein and electrolyte content, causing mucoviscidosis.

A sodium content above 100 mmol/L is consistent with the diagnosis. Direct measurement of the immunoglobulins would exclude hypogammaglobulinaemia. Other investigations include an assessment of pancreatic exocrine function. An oral glucose tolerance test is useful to assess endocrine pancreatic function.

Cystic fibrosis is an autosomal recessive condition caused by mutations of a gene located on the long arm of chromosome 7. This encodes the cystic fibrosis transmembrane conductance regulator (CFTR) that is involved in the transport of electrolytes across cell membranes.

The condition is characterized by abnormal exocrine secretion. The major clinical features include chronic pulmonary disease, pancreatic dysfunction resulting in malabsorption, poor growth and diabetes mellitus. The most important problems are respiratory: recurrent bronchiolar obstruction causes bronchiectasis, atelectasis and chronic infection which gradually destroys lung function, ultimately leading to pulmonary insufficiency, and cor pulmonale. Allergic bronchopulmonary aspergillosis is common. The lungs often become colonized by *Staphylococcus pyogenes* and *Pseudomonas aeruginosa*. Hypoplasia of the gall bladder occurs and there is an increased tendency to form gallstones; blockage of bile ducts leads to pericholangitis, periportal fibrosis and biliary cirrhosis. Intestinal problems are related to the secretion of abnormal amounts of viscid mucus and include meconium ileus, intestinal obstruction and reduced transit in the distal bowel.

Treatment is partially successful so that patients now regularly reach adulthood. Physiotherapy and replacement of pancreatic enzymes are the two principal measures. Immunization and the rapid use of antibiotics help to minimize pulmonary damage. Ranitidine is helpful in decreasing the acid digestion of pancreatic enzymes. Genetic counselling should be offered to the parents and other unaffected siblings; prenatal diagnosis is now available.

Other notes
- In hypogammaglobulinaemia there is a normal albumin and a low protein level due to low immunoglobulins. While children have recurrent childhood infections, they rarely fail to thrive.
- Coeliac disease causes low vitamin B_{12}, folate and iron. It is not classically associated with steatorrhoea, and is not associated with bronchiectasis.

Answer to question 95

a) 2. Coronary artery disease of the left anterior descending artery.

ST segment depression extending from lead V3 to V6 of more than 2 mm suggests ischaemia in the region supplied by the left anterior descending artery.

b) 4. Aortic stenosis.

The QRS complexes in the V leads demonstrate the voltage criteria for left ventricular hypertrophy. In the absence of systemic hypertension, aortic stenosis must be considered. This may cause exercise-induced ischaemia without coronary artery disease.

An echocardiogram is required to exclude aortic stenosis. A coronary angiogram should be carried out to assess the extent of coronary artery disease.

a) 2. Secondary syphilis (*Treponema pallidum*).

b) 1. Membranous glomerulonephritis.

The features suggesting a diagnosis of secondary syphilis are the characteristic rash associated with lymphadenopathy and painless mucosal ulceration. The combination of peripheral oedema and heavy proteinuria suggest that he has developed a nephrotic syndrome.

Nephrotic syndrome can occur as a result of a wide variety of systemic diseases, including diabetes mellitus, systemic lupus erythematosus and amyloidosis. Drugs and malignancies, particularly lymphoma, are other well-recognized precipitants. Infectious causes include hepatitis B and C, HIV and syphilis.

The most common histological lesions associated with primary nephrotic syndrome in adults are in order of frequency: membranous glomerulo-nephropathy, focal segmental glomerulosclerosis and minimal change disease; and more rarely, membranoproliferative glomerulonephritis.

T. pallidum is the bacterium that causes venereal syphilis. There had been a steady decline in the incidence of syphilis, but numbers are now increasing and the diagnosis should be considered in patients with HIV infection, the sexually promiscuous and in immigrants from eastern Europe.

- Primary infection leads to a sore at the site of inoculation and this is usually on the genitalia. Typically this would present 3 weeks after contact and then gradually heal. Patients may then develop a secondary stage characterized by a generalized symmetrical painless, non-itchy rash. Infection may then become dormant. Tertiary syphilis may then occur and involves the skin mucous membranes and bones. In more severe cases it will also affect the central nervous system, aorta and other internal organs.
- Treatment is with high dose penicillin. The Jarisch–Herxheimer reaction can complicate treatment. This is due to the release of endotoxin-like substances when large numbers of the bacterium are killed after the initiation of antibiotics.

Diagnosis

The diagnosis is made by combining clinical features with corresponding serology (see the following box and tables). Treponemes can be visualized with direct phase contrast or dark backround microscopy but this can be insensitive because lesions often contain relatively few organisms and active disease may only be transient.

Common clinical features associated with syphilis

Primary infection
- A painless papule with rapid ulceration (chancre) is present, usually on the penis, or more commonly the rectum in the homosexual male.

Secondary infection
- There is a symmetrical non-irritating rash with generalized painless lymphadenopathy. The rash is also present on the hands and feet.
- Papules may enlarge in moist areas such as the perineum, genitalia and under the breasts to form condylomata lata (these are very infectious).
- Mucous patches in the mouth form grayish erosions and these are called 'snail track ulcers'.

Tertiary infection
- **Neurosyphilis** can lead to almost any neurological sequelae. The most common manifestations are related to dorsal column loss (tabes dorsalis) and dementia (general paralysis of the insane (GPI) and meningovascular involvement.
- **Cardiovascular** syphilis is characterized by an aortitis, which usually involves the aortic root but may affect other parts of the aorta. The most frequent clinical manifestations of aortitis associated with late syphilis are aortic regurgitation, aortic aneurysm and angina.
- **Gummata** are inflammatory fibrous nodules or plaques, which can occur in any organ but most often affect the skin and bone. Cutaneous gummas are multiple painless nodules, which can break down and form ulcers. Mucosal gummas seen in the oropharynx and nasal septum lead to ulceration and local destruction. Syphilis of the bones leads to an osteoperostitis and leads to bone pain, particularly at night.

Answer to question 96 continued overleaf

Summary of serological markers for syphilis						
Diagnosis	VDRL	Titre	TPHA	FTA — Abs		Comments
				IgG	IgM	
Early untreated primary syphilis	+ or −	Rising	+ or −	+	+	FTA – Abs is the first test to become +. VDRL − in 30% of cases
Untreated late, primary or secondary syphilis or reinfection	+	High or rising	+	+	+	
Untreated latent syphilis	+ or −	Moderate	+	+	+	
Biological false positive reaction	+	Low	−	−	−	FTA – Abs may be weakly positive

Results positive	Diagnosis
None	Syphilis not present or very early infection
All	Untreated, recently treated or latent syphilis
VDRL and FTA	Primary syphilis
TPHA and FTA	Treated syphilis or untreated latent or late
FTA only	Early primary syphilis – untreated or recently treated early syphilis
TPHA only	Treated syphilis
VDRL only	False positive reaction

1. Commence nifedipine.

The main determinants of aortic regurgitant volume are the orifice area, the duration of diastole (a function of heart rate) and the diastolic transvalvular pressure gradient (aortic minus left ventricular diastolic pressure).

- Treating hypertension and avoiding bradycardia is therefore desirable.

Aortic regurgitation leads to volume overload on the left ventricle; left ventricular dilatation and hypertrophy result. Arteriolar vasodilators redistribute left ventricular stroke volume by increasing forward flow and reducing regurgitant flow. Venodilators and diuretics will diminish preload and will reduce both left ventricular end diastolic volume and pressure. They can therefore be used to alleviate signs and symptoms of heart failure and preserve left ventricular function by reducing wall stress.

Nifedipine has been shown to reduce symptoms and mortality most effectively in asymptomatic patients awaiting valve repair. Limited trials of ACEIs in this setting have been inconsistent.

a) 3. Systemic sclerosis.

The diagnosis is progressive systemic sclerosis. Raynaud's phenomenon, pruritus, prolonged tanning and skin oedema are common features of early progressive systemic sclerosis. As the disease progresses, major organs become involved, particularly the lungs, kidneys, gut and heart.

b) 1, 3, 6. Interstitial pneumonitis, pulmonary hypertension, renovascular disease.

Interstitial pneumonitis: she has shortness of breath on exertion, basal crackles and pulmonary function tests consistent with lung restriction (loss of lung volume and a reduced TLCO). Pulmonary manifestations, including interstitial pneumonitis, pulmonary fibrosis, pleural thickening and pleural effusions, are common in progressive systemic sclerosis and may occur early.

Pulmonary hypertension: progressive interstitial lung disease may be complicated by pulmonary hypertension and right-sided heart failure, a frequent cause of death in progressive systemic sclerosis. Pulmonary hypertension secondary to an extensive pulmonary artery sclerosis may occur in the absence of pulmonary fibrosis. Treatment of interstitial pneumonitis and progressive lung fibrosis is immunosuppression with prednisolone and cytotoxic agents such as cyclophosphamide. A rare pulmonary complication of progressive systemic sclerosis is alveolar cell or bronchiolar carcinoma.

Renovascular disease (renal scleroderma crisis): she has developed a renal scleroderma crisis – her blood pressure and her plasma creatinine levels are elevated (taking into consideration her age and urea level). Renovascular hypertension is generally a late but ominous complication of progressive systemic sclerosis, often leading to rapidly progressive and irreversible renal failure. The onset of the hypertension is often sudden and may be heralded by headaches. Urgent control of the blood pressure as an inpatient is indicated, using intravenous prostaglandins and an ACE inhibitor. Often, even with control of the blood pressure, renal function continues to decline and some patients will require a period of dialysis. Patients on corticosteroids appear to be more likely to present with malignant hypertension. If a patient with systemic sclerosis needs to be on steroids then they should also be on an ACE inhibitor.

a) 3. Chronic lymphatic leukaemia with autoimmune haemolytic anaemia.

b) 3. Direct Coombs' test.

The presence of lymphocytosis with lymphadenopathy and splenomegaly in this age group is very suggestive of chronic lymphatic leukaemia. Anaemia in chronic lymphatic leukaemia may be caused by marrow infiltration, hypersplenism or an autoimmune haemolytic anaemia. In this patient the polychromasia, spherocytosis, reticulocytosis and absent haptoglobins point to a diagnosis of haemolysis. Acute myeloid leukaemia may present with a pancytopenia; the white cell count may be high or low but the number of lymphocytes would not be expected. A haemolytic anaemia is not characteristic of acute myeloid leukaemia although note that patients with acute promyelocytic M3 subtypes can present with disseminated intravascular coagulation.

About 20% of patients with chronic lymphatic leukaemia will develop a positive Coombs' test at some time during their illness but only one-third will develop significant haemolysis. The haemolysis responds well to steroids and chlorambucil.

Chronic lymphocytic anaemia accounts for 70% of lymphocytic leukaemias; patients are typically between 60 and 80 years of age. They usually present incidentally with a lymphocytosis; others may present with lymphadenopathy or symptoms of anaemia. Splenomegaly is found in 50%. A lymphocytosis $>10 \times 10^9/L$ is required for diagnosis in conjunction with >30% lymphocytes in bone marrow aspirates. Immunophenotyping can be used to diagnose patients outside of these criteria.

The course and prognosis of lymphocytic leukaemia is very variable and patients are staged according to the degree of anaemia, thrombocytopenia, palpable nodes and organomegaly. Further prognostic factors include the response to therapy, the lymphocyte doubling time and the underlying chromosomal abnormalities.

Complications include infections – pneumonia is the leading cause of death. Autoimmune haemolytic anaemia is also well recognized and produces a positive direct antiglobulin Coombs' test.

a) 3. Mitral stenosis.

This M-mode clearly cuts across the mitral valve, which is thickened and shows the seperation of the anterior and posterior leaflets. **Rheumatic fever** is the only common cause of mitral stenosis.

Structure A is the intraventricular septum. The right ventricle is above and the left ventricle below the line.

b) 4. Posterior leaflet mitral valve.

The two leaflets of the mitral valve separate in diastole; their echo signal is normally a sharp single line each, and they move in opposite directions. B is the posterior leaflet and (i) is thickened, and (ii) moves anteriorly in diastole (i.e. upwards). This is characteristic of mitral stenosis. In addition the normal pattern of movement of the leaflets is to drift together in mid-diastole and to re-open with atrial contraction. When the left atrial pressure is high they remain open at the limit of their excursion at all times, as shown here.

c) 4. Opening snap.

With a mobile stenosed valve, mitral valve opening can be heard as an early diastolic opening snap. This occurs at line C.

a) 4. Avascular necrosis of the femoral head.

Other joints that can be affected are the head of the humerus, medial and lateral condyles of the distal femur and the superior margin of the talus.

b) 3. Plain X-rays of the hips.

The plain X-ray is often initially normal but may show an infarcted area with surrounding radiolucency, a sclerotic rim around the lesion, loose fragments of bone, or fractures. If the plain X-rays are normal then MRI is the investigation of choice and is sensitive enough to detect the changes of avascular necrosis which may not be seen on either plain X-rays or on an isotope bone scan. An isotope bone scan, which is likely to be more readily available, will initially show an area of reduced uptake which may be surrounded by increased tracer localization. As repair gets under way, or if there is extensive damage (e.g. with a fracture) there may be generally increased uptake.

High dose steroids are the most important cause of osteonecrosis, and in this patient, may have contributed both directly and indirectly by causing weight gain.

The patient received a huge excess of dexamethasone (approximately equivalent to 150 mg hydrocortisone per day). Replacement regimens of hydrocortisone vary from 20–30 mg per day.

Factors implicated in the pathogenesis of osteonecrosis include:
1. Trauma, e.g. fracture
2. Excess corticosteroids
3. Sickle cell disease
4. Deep-sea diving
5. Radiotherapy
6. Alcohol
7. Pregnancy
8. Rheumatic diseases, e.g. rheumatoid arthritis, systemic lupus erythematosus
9. Hereditary disorders, e.g. Fabry's disease, Gaucher's disease, hyperlipidaemia
10. Infection, e.g. infective endocarditis
11. Idiopathic, e.g. Perthe's disease.

a) 3. Acute thyrotoxicosis.

b) 3. IV carbimazole.

4. IV beta blockers.

There is a family history of autoimmune disease and a good history of progressive weight loss – an indication of hyperthyroidism. The acute deterioration followed an upper respiratory tract infection and the patient presented with the classic combination of: (i) fever; (ii) cardiovascular symptoms – arrhythmias and hypotension; (iii) neurological involvement – confusion, agitation; (iv) gastrointestinal involvement with abdominal pain and vomiting.

Acute thyrotoxicosis is a medical emergency. The immediate management steps are:

- Intravenous beta blockers – propranolol 2 mg IV is effective in relieving fever and tachycardia.
- 20 mg of carbimazole **orally** or by nasogastric tube, repeated 4-hourly, or an equivalent dosage of propylthiouracil (these preparations cannot be given intravenously.)
- In some centres, sodium iodide is given 1 h after the first dose of carbimazole to prevent further release of thyroid hormones.
- Hydrocortisone should be administered 200 mg IV, then 100mg 8-hourly.
- General supportive treatment should include intravenous fluids; the patient may need appropriate sedation and digoxin may be necessary to control the atrial fibrillation. Active cooling should be instituted (aspirin should be avoided as an antipyretic because it displaces thyroid hormone from thyroid-binding globulin).
- Blood should be sent for measurement of thyroid hormones and thyroid autoantibodies.

A

a) 2. Haemophilia A.
b) 2. Prolonged bleeding 3. Recurrent haemarthroses.

The coagulation tests show a prolonged activated partial thromboplastin time (APTT) but normal prothrombin time (PT), indicating an abnormality of the intrinsic pathway of coagulation. The bleeding time is normal. The commonest cause of such an abnormality is factor VIII:C deficiency – **haemophilia A**, an X-linked recessive condition.
Factor IX deficiency – haemophilia B/Christmas disease (X-linked recessive) will also produce the same abnormal clotting profile but its incidence is one-fifth that of haemophilia A.

Prolonged bleeding and **recurrent haemarthrosis:** severe factor VIII:C deficiency (<1% normal levels) causes impaired generation of thrombin and results in bleeding into major weight-bearing joints and prolonged bleeding after surgery or dental extraction. Intracranial bleeding is the commonest cause of death in severe untreated haemophilia; other common sites of bleeding include the renal tract, muscles, subperiosteal region and the iliopsoas sheath. The severity of symptoms depends on the extent of factor VIII:C deficiency.

Primary haemostasis, which is caused by a combination of vasoconstriction and platelet aggregation, is normal in haemophilia A and B and there is no abnormality in the initial haemostatic response. The diagnosis may be confirmed by demonstrating a deficiency of factor VIII:C and normal levels of factor IX and X.

Other notes
- In von Willebrand's disease (autosomal dominant inheritance) abnormal platelet function is associated with low factor VIII:C and VIIIR:AG activity. The following tests are abnormal: prolonged APTT (may be normal), prolonged bleeding time and impaired ristocetin-induced platelet aggregation.
- The coagulation screen:
  - **The activated partial thromboplastic time (APTT)** (30–46 s) measures the intrinsic clotting system and the 'common pathway' of the clotting cascade where prothrombin is activated to thrombin. The APTT is prolonged by abnormalities of plasma factors II, V, VIII, IX, X, XI, XII and by extrinsic inhibitors such as heparin.
  - **The prothrombin time** (PT) (10–14 s). This is prolonged with deficiencies of plasma factors II, V, VII, X and fibrinogen. It is also used to measure the inhibition of the vitamin K dependent clotting cascade by warfarin – this is expressed as a ratio compared to a normal control (INR).

- **The bleeding time** can evaluate overall platelet function as well as number. The usual bleeding time is between 4 and 7 min. It will be prolonged if the platelet count falls to below $50 \times 10^9/L$. In von Willebrand's disease the bleeding is usually prolonged as a result of a decrease or abnormality of the plasma von Willebrand factor which is involved in the binding of platelets to matrix proteins and other cells.

1. Start perindopril 2 mg.

Calcific **aortic stenosis** may be caused by progressive calcification of a congenitally bicuspid valve typically presenting in the 4th to 5th decade. Senile calcification of a normal valve presents later. Rheumatic disease of the aortic valve usually causes mixed stenotic and regurgitent lesions and is commonly associated with mitral valve disease.

Cardiac output is maintained at the cost of an increasing gradient across the valve. There is left ventricular hypertrophy and coronary blood flow might be inadequate.

The fixed outflow obstruction negates the required increase in cardiac output required with exercise and effort-related syncope can occur. With increasing stenosis, then, the left ventricle will fail and patients tend to deteriorate rapidly.

Management is surgical and aortic valve repair is the commonest valve replacement in the West.

Beta blockers and nitrates can be used sparingly and may control hypertension and angina. Nitrates can often lead to symptomatic hypotension. Diuretics are often prescribed for acute pulmonary oedema but patients often rely on adequate filling pressures to maintain cardiac output – excessive treatment may therefore be hazardous.

ACEIs are traditionally avoided because of the ensuing hypotension. Recent small trials have shown that very cautious introduction in the hospital can be effective.

By comparison in **mitral stenosis,** the flow of blood from the left atrium to the left ventricle is severely impeded leading to pulmonary congestion and breathlessness. There is dilatation and hypertrophy of the left atrium. Left ventricular filling becomes more dependent on left atrial contraction. Any increase in heart rate shortens diastole (and the time that the mitral valve is open) and produces a further rise in left atrial pressure. Situations that demand an increase in cardiac output will also increase left atrial pressure. Exercise and pregnancy are therefore poorly tolerated.

Atrial fibrillation caused by progressive dilatation of the left ventricle is the commonest complication and has a high chance of embolism. Early treatment is recommended in any patient who has atrial fibrillation or evidence of an embolus.

The onset of atrial fibrillation is associated with a dramatic reduction in left ventricular filling: Good rate control with digoxin, beta blockers and rate-limiting calcium antagonists is therefore necessary.

a) 3. Normal pressure hydrocephalus.

b) 3. Ventricular peritoneal shunt.

Normal pressure hydrocephalus can be considered to be a triad of amnesia (often with psychomotor retardation), progressive gait disability (small tottering steps) and urinary incontinence.

- The onset is typically insidious but may be rapid.
- There is dilatation of the cerebral ventricles caused by subarachnoid obstruction but normal cerebrospinal fluid pressure is recorded if a lumbar puncture is performed.
- The syndrome has been observed following head injury, subarachnoid haemorrhage, intracranial surgery, cerebrovascular disease and meningoencephalitis, and in association with lesions that obstruct the 3rd ventricle such as gliomas, cerebellar haemangioblastomas, aqueduct stenosis, 3rd ventricular cysts, and aberrant blood vessels. In 50% of cases there is no clear cause.
- There is impaired outflow and resorption of cerebrospinal fluid; this dilates the ventricles, stretches the periventricular pathways, reduces cerebral blood flow and causes oedema of the periventricular substance.
- Positron-emission tomography has demonstrated generalized disturbances of cerebral metabolism in normal pressure hydrocephalus as distinct from degenerative diseases.
- Cerebrospinal fluid diversion procedures in selected patients can completely reverse the abnormalities (generally ventriculoatrial or ventriculo-peritoneal shunts).
- It is important to distinguish normal pressure hydrocephalus from the passive ventricular enlargement secondary to cerebral atrophy, which will not benefit from a shunt procedure.
- CT scanning and intracranial pressure measurement are useful – lack of cortical atrophy and the presence of frontal white matter and periventricular lucency favour normal pressure hydrocephalus.
- Cerebrospinal fluid diversion may be complicated by shunt infection, subdural haematomas, epilepsy, and malfunction.

2. 50%.

Dystrophin gene deletions are tested for with the use of DNA-based technology when the clinical symptoms and signs suggest the diagnosis. In this case the test can be performed because the brother has been found to have Duchenne's muscular dystrophy (DMD).

Note: a negative test can occur in 30% of patients with DMD – some mutations are not detected by current DNA testing. A muscle biopsy is therefore required in cases of uncertainty.

DMD is an X-linked recessive condition causing progressive skeletal muscle weakness and cardiomyopathy. Affected children are usually unable to walk by 12 years. Death is due to progressive cardiomyopathy or respiratory failure.
The daughter has a 50% chance of being a carrier.

a) 5. C1-esterase inhibitor deficiency

b) 3. *Streptococcus milleri.*

The history of recurrent chest infections is strongly suggestive of bronchiectasis. Cystic fibrosis would be top of the list of differential diagnoses. An underlying pathological cause for bronchiectasis can be found in 40% of cases.

Causes of bronchiectasis

Immune deficiency
- Panhypoglobulinaemia
- Selective immunoglobulin deficiency

Excessive immune response
- Allergic bronchopulmonary aspergillosis

Mucocillary clearance defects
- Kartageners syndrome[a]
- Cystic fibrosis
- Young's syndrome[b]

Toxic insults
- Aspiration of gastric contents

Mechanical obstruction
- Intrinsic tumours and foreign bodies

Post infective
- Whooping cough
- Persistant childhood infections
- Tuberculosis

[a]Kartagener's syndrome: triad of sinusitis, situs inversus and bronchiectasis
[b]Young's syndrome: obstructive azoospermia and bronchiectasis

Organisms commonly recovered from the sputum in a patient with bronchiectasis due to cystic fibrosis would include:
- *Pseudomonas aeruginosa* and the mucoid variant would be considered virtually pathognomonic of cystic fibrosis
- Gram-negative bacteria such as *E. coli*, *Proteus* and *Klebsiella*
- *Haemophilus influenza* and *Staphylococcus aureus*
- *Aspergillus fumigatus* and *Candida*.

4. Buerger's disease (thromboangiitis obliterans).

This does not occur exclusively in males. Patients from southern Europe can be amongst the heaviest smokers in the world and many smoke unfiltered cigarettes with a high tar content.

Thromboangiitis obliterans is an inflammatory occlusive peripheral vascular disease of unknown aetiology that affects medium-sized arteries and veins. It occurs more commonly in males and almost exclusively in smokers.

The clinical features of thomboangiitis obliterans include a triad of claudication, Raynaud's phenomenon and a migratory superficial vein thrombophebitis.
- Claudication most commonly occurs in the calves, feet, forearms and hands, reflecting the distal distribution of disease.
- Gangrene occurs at the finger tips due to digitial ischaemia.
- Brachial and popliteal pulses are present but radial, ulnar and tibial pulse can be absent.

Doppler ultrasound will demonstrate absent peripheral pulses and digital subtraction angiography will show the characteristic 'corkscrew' collaterals.

There is no specific treatment except abstention from tobacco. Vascular perfusion improves when individuals are no longer exposed to cigarettes. With acute ischaemia, intravenous prostacyclin and oral aspirin may help.

Other notes
- The patient needs a blood film, iron studies and haemoglobin electrophoresis. Her microcytic anaemia may be due to iron deficiency secondary to menorrhagia. If the patient is shown to be deficent in iron, gastrointestinal examination with an upper gastrointestinal endoscopy and colonoscopy should be considered at this stage.
- Thalassaemia trait is a common cause of a microcytic anaemia in a Mediterranean patient.
- The elevated CRP is due to infection.
- Cryoglobulinaemia is very unlikely as the complement levels are normal (this is classically associated with a low C4 and normal C3).
- Involvement of the upper and lower limbs makes cholesterol emboli very unlikely.

3. Leucopenia secondary to azathioprine.

The patient has developed an acute bacterial pneumonia and is markedly leucopenic. The most likely explanation is that he has been prescribed allopurinol for his gout. This is a xanthine oxidase inhibitor and has resulted in the development of azathioprine toxicity leading to bone marrow suppression, leucopenia and acute sepsis.

Azathioprine is a prodrug and is converted to 6-mercaptopurine. 6 mercaptopurine is then converted to thiopurine nucleotides which decrease de novo purine synthesis and are incorporated into native nucleic acid resulting in cytotoxicity and decreased cellular proliferation.

6-mercaptopurine is metabolized by two enzymes, xanthine oxidase and thiopurine methyl transferase, to inactive metabolites. Blacks have lower thiopurine transferase levels than whites. Ninety percent of whites have high levels, 10% have intermediate levels and 0.3% have low levels.

Patients with constitutively low thiopurine methyl transferase levels are at risk of bone marrow suppression (at 4–10 weeks) if prescribed azathioprine. Inhibition of xanthine oxidase levels by allopurinol or of thiopurine methyltransferase by sulphasalazine results in accumulation of 6 mercaptopurine and toxicity. If allopurinol is coprescribed with azathioprine the dose of the latter should be reduced by 75%.

Emergency therapy for the patient's pneumonia is needed, with hydration, oxygen, bronchodilators and broad spectrum antibiotics. Allopurinol should be stopped, and it would be acutely advisable to stop the azathioprine. Colony-stimulating factors may be useful in drug-induced leukopenia in patients whose marrow is slow to recover and who have life-threatening sepsis.

3. She needs a tissue valve replacement.

With an aortic valve gradient of 70 mmHg this lady has severe aortic stenosis. Valve replacement is required. The life of a tissue valve is limited and therefore, in this age group, a metal valve would be recommended, however, this clearly has implications in pregnancy because she would require lifelong warfarinization. The management of choice would therefore be to give a prosthetic valve during her reproductive years.

2. Institute insulin – dextrose sliding scale.

The DIGAMI (Diabetes Mellitus Insulin Glucose Infusion In Acute Myocardial Infarction) trial provided clear evidence that mortality in diabetic patients who have myocardial infarction is reduced by the immediate use of insulin and glucose infusion followed by a multidose insulin regimen. There is a 1-year decrease in mortality of 30% and an 11% reduction in mortality over 3.6 years. In the DIGAMI study, patients were enrolled who had had an acute myocardial infarction within the preceeding 24 h combined with previously known diabetes mellitus and a blood glucose concentration >11 mmol/L, or a similar blood glucose concentration without known diabetes mellitus. Patients received an insulin-glucose infusion for at least 24 h. This was followed by sc insulin 4 times daily for at least 3 months.

Patients were previously untreated with insulin and with a comparatively low risk profile (age <70 and with no previous cardiac history). This effect may be related to reduced ischaemic injury during the acute phase, protecting against further myocardial dysfunction. Intense insulin treatment may help to restore impaired platelet function, correct the disturbed lipoprotein pattern and decrease plasma activity of plasminogen activator inhibitor, which is high in diabetic patients.

*Note: despite such impressive results the DIGAMI study was not a randomized controlled trial; there is also a suggestion that the results might have been attributable to the closer attention given to tighter insulin control and that the same benefits could be gained with oral agents. These questions are likely to be addressed with further trials in this area.

A **beta blocker** would be relatively contraindicated given the history of asthma.

Other notes
- **Glycoprotein IIb/IIIa** inhibitors prevent platelet aggregation by blocking the binding of fibrinogen to receptors on platelets. Abciximab is a monoclonal antibody which binds principally to glycoprotein IIb/IIIa receptors. It is licensed for use in conjunction with heparin and aspirin for the prevention of ischaemic complications in high-risk patients undergoing percutaneous transluminal coronary angiography.
  Eptifibatide and tirofibran also inhibit glycoprotein IIb/IIIa receptors. They are licensed for use with heparin and aspirin to prevent early myocardial infarction in patients with unstable angina or non Q wave myocardial infarction.
- A **statin** would be indicated in this patient post-myocardial infarction.
  Multiple secondary prevention trials have demonstrated the benefit of lowering lipid levels in patients with coronary disease. This benefit has been shown in post-myocardial infarction patients with marked hyper-cholesteraemia as well as those with high, mildly elevated and more recently normal lipid levels. There is also an increasing indication that statins (HMG Co A reductase inhibitors) have an antiinflammatory property as well as favourable effects on endothelial function.

4. Conn's syndrome.

The most marked abnormality on the ECG is the presence of inverted ST segments and U waves: These are associated with hypokalaemia.

The U wave is a short upstroke that follows the T wave: it represents part of the repolarization process and is best seen in V2–V4. The U wave can be normal in the anterior leads if the T waves are not flattened. Other common causes of U waves are:
- Hypomagnesaemia
- Hypocalcaemia
- Hypothyroidism.

Characteristics of hypokalaemia on ECG
- Prolongs the QT interval (measured from the onset of the QRS to the end of the T wave and corrected for rate, but any QT interval longer then 440 ms (11 small squares) is probably pathological.)
- The T wave might be flattened and followed by a U wave
- The PR interval might be prolonged
- The ST segments might be depressed

Remember that **Conn's syndrome** or primary hyperaldosteronism is a cause of secondary hypertension. Primary hyperaldosteronism may be caused by:
- A single adenoma in the adrenal in 50% of cases
- Multiple adenomata in 10% of cases
- Bilateral nodules in the remainder.

Aldosterone enhances sodium and hence water reabsorption from the distal tubule in exchange for hydrogen or potassium ions, resulting in intravascular volume expansion and a **hypokalaemic alkalosis.**

The diagnosis would be confirmed with high aldosterone levels in the presence of low renin levels. Further imaging or selective venous catheterization may then be used to locate the source.

The voltage criteria for left ventricular hypertrophy are that the normal height of the R wave in V5 or V6 added to the depth of the S wave in V2 is greater then 35 mm (some recommend adding the greatest positive and negative deflections). However, this measurement can be variable. These limits are often exceeded in young fit individuals.

3. Combined amitriptyline and ethylene glycol overdose.

Although he seems to have taken an amitriptyline overdose he also has a profound raised **anion gap metabolic acidosis**. The anion gap can be estimated with the following formula:

anion gap = sodium + potassium − [chloride + bicarbonate]

The normal range is 7–17 mmol/L. The anion gap in this patient is 34.8 mmol/L. The causes of a raised anion gap associated with a metabolic acidosis include:

- Renal failure
- Ketoacidosis
- Methanol/ethylene glycol
- Salicylate poisoning
- Lactic acidosis.

Ethylene glycol toxicity causes a profound anion gap metabolic acidosis and a raised osmolar gap.

- Ethylene glycol undergoes hepatic degradation by alcohol dehydrogenase with the production of toxic metabolites that lead to an acidosis.
- Oxalic acid is also precipitated as calcium oxalate crystals in the renal tubules rapidly leading to renal failure.
- Oxalate crystals can therefore be detected in the urine (this patient has crystalluria).
- Toxicity is characterized initially by inebriation, ataxia and metabolic acidosis with respiratory compensation, seizures and hypocalcaemia (this must be monitored carefully during treatment).
- 12–30 h after ingestion, respiratory function usually deteriorates and there may be cardiorespiratory failure.
- In patients who survive this period, renal failure usually develops.
- Ethanol competitively inhibits the breakdown of ethylene glycol into toxic metabolites and may therefore be given as a 10% ethanol infusion. Fomepizole an inhibitor of alcohol dehydrogenase may also be used. Sodium bicarbonate can also be given to normalize the pH.
- Haemodialysis is the definitive treatment for both ethylene glycol and methanol poisoning. They both have a low level of protein binding, low volume of distribution and high water solubility. Indications include levels greater then 50mg/dL, profound metabolic acidosis, renal failure and evidence of early visual symptoms that are characteristic of a severe methanol overdose.

Tricyclic antidepressant (TCA) overdoses account for the largest percentage of deaths caused by pharmacological agents in suicide attempts.

- TCAs produce anticholinergic effects consisting of:
  1. Hypotension
  2. Sinus tachycardia
  3. Pupil dilation

4. Dry mouth, respiratory depression

5. Ileus and urinary retention

6. Ventricular arrythmias and conduction abnormalities can occur up to 24 h after ingestion. ECG changes include prolongation of the PR and QT intervals, widening of the QRS interval or the appearance of bundle branch block.

- Treatment is with sodium bicarbonate sufficient to raise the pH to above 7.5. This increases protein binding of the drug which is pH dependent; the extracellular load also increases sodium channel function.
- Activated charcoal may be given.
- Forced diuresis, or haemodialysis play no part in drug removal (they are lipophilic and 98% protein bound).

3. Acute myelomonocytic leukaemia (M4).

The most likely diagnosis is acute myeloid leukaemia (AML). This is accountable for 80% of acute leukaemia in adults. It is more common in men then women and often presents in the 6th and 7th decades. Gingival hyperplasia is commonly seen in myelomonocytic (M4) and monocytic (M5) subtypes of AML.

AML is a disease of immature haematopoetic cells. The proliferating cells predominate in the bone marrow and replace other haematopoetic elements. Patients often present with infections, anaemia or bleeding complications.

Congenital disorders such as Down's syndrome can predispose to developing AML. High dose radiation, chronic benzene exposure and alkylating agents have also been associated.

Generally, patients have an absence of clinical features. Splenomegaly is present in 20%.

Patients with AML are anaemic and pancytopenic: anaemia is the most constant finding and it is usually normochromic and normocytic. Reticulocyte counts are usually low. The white cell count may be low or very high (from 1×10^9/L to 200×10^9/L). Examination reveals the presence of blast cells. Auer rods are stick-like cytoplasmic inclusions that are diagnostic and they are seen in 20% of patients; they are often better seen in bone marrow samples.

AML can be classified into subtypes M0–M7. This is based on cell morphology, histochemical stains and cell surface markers. Some subtypes have notable clinical features, e.g. acute promyelocytic subtype M3 is often associated with disseminated intravascular coagulation, whereas acute myelomonocytic (M4) and acute monocytic (M5) subtypes commonly involve abnormalities in the extramedullary tissues – the skin, gingival and nervous system.

Patients with any acute leukaemia require both supportive care and consideration of appropriate chemotherapy.

Supportive therapy includes prophylactic platelet transfusions if the platelet count is <10×10^9/L. Clotting abnormalities require correction. Patients require close montoring for signs of infection with early institution of intravenous broad spectrum antimicrobial agents.

The aim of chemotherapy is to introduce remission and maintain this with further courses of consolidation therapy to eradicate the leukaemic cell population. Up to 85% of patients who achieve a complete remission will relapse. Transplantation reduces relapse risk but has high procedural mortality.

Factors associated with a poor prognosis in AML are age over 60 years and a presenting white cell count of >50×10^9/L. Other features include the presence of blasts in cerebrospinal fluid and >20% of blasts in the fluid after initial chemotherapy. Deletions of chromosomes 5 and 7 also confer a poor prognosis. A patient with AML aged over 60 years has a 10% chance of surviving for 5 years.

Answer to question 115

a) 3. Primary hyperaldosteronism (Conn's syndrome).

b) 4. Serum aldosterone and renin (supine samples).

This occurs due to an adrenal adenoma or adrenal hyperplasia. The combination of hypertension with the biochemical picture of hypernatraemia, hypokalaemia and a high serum bicarbonate concentration is typical. The endocrinological diagnosis is confirmed by high serum aldosterone levels in the presence of low renin levels. The hypertension is typically resistant to ACE inhibitors. Arteriography and venous sampling, CT scanning, and cholesterol scanning are used to localize the source of aldosterone prior to surgery.

Other notes
- Phaeochromocytoma is characterized by episodic hypertension, hyperglycaemia and weight loss. Periods of crisis are characterized by fever, headache, palpitations, sweating and nausea. Investigations include 24-h urinary cateocholamines and MIBG scan.
- Hypertension and a hypokalaemic alkalosis are also seen with ectopic ACTH production but the glucose level is usually elevated.

a) 4. Axonal neuropathy.

b) 3. Isoniazid induced.

An isoniazid drug administered as part of the patient's anti-tuberculous chemotherapy regimen, is the most likely cause.

An axonal neuropathy is characterized by diminution of the action potential with normal conduction velocity.

The most useful information from the analysis of the nerve conduction studies is the conduction speed and the amplitude of the waveform. The amplitude reflects the total number of fibres stimulated whilst the conduction velocity is the function of the largest nerve fibres that have the most myelin and the longest internode length. Usually conduction velocities are greater than 50m/s in the arms and greater than 40m/s in the legs.

With axonal neuropathies there is reduction in amplitude of the CMAP (compound muscle action potential) in the motor nerve conduction and of the CNAP (compound nerve action potential) in the sensory and mixed nerve conduction in the presence of near normal nerve conduction velocities, and of normal duration and shape of the CMAP and CNAP.

With demyelination one sees slowing of conduction velocity with conduction block and abnormal temporal dispersion.

Other causes of an axonal neuropathy
- Alcohol
- Vasculitis
- Acute axonal neuropathy
- Drugs and toxins, e.g. arsenic
- Diabetes
- Uraemia
- Vitamin B_{12} deficiency
- Folic acid deficiency
- Hypothyroidism
- Malignancy

Causes of demyelinating neuropathy
- Guillaine–Barré syndrome
- HIV
- Diptheria
- Acute inflammatory demyelinating polyneuropathy
- Chronic inflammatory demyelinating polyneuropathy
- Monoclonal gammopathy
- Hereditary sensory motor neuropathy, e.g. Charcot–Marie–Tooth disease
- Diabetes
- Hypothyroidism

Answer to question 117

a) 1. Oral propanolol.

b) 3. Secondary to cirrhosis.

Portal hypertension arises due to an increased resistance to portal blood flow. The causes may be divided broadly into three groups:
1. Prehepatic, e.g. portal vein thrombosis
2. Hepatic: (a) presinusoidal (e.g. schistosomiasis), (b) sinusoidal (e.g. cirrhosis)
3. Post hepatic, e.g. Budd Chiari syndrome, constrictive pericarditis

As a consequence of portal hypertension, collateral vessels form between portal and systemic vessels, with the most important clinical consequence being bleeding from gastrointestinal varices. There are a number of treatment options:
- Propanolol is the mainstay of treatment for primary prophylaxis against variceal bleeding, lowering the risk of bleeding but not affecting overall mortality. It achieves a reduction in the portal pressure gradient by causing splanchnic vasoconstriction and reducing cardiac output.
- Isosorbide mononitrate may be used in those patients where beta blockers are contraindicated.
- Sclerotherapy is not beneficial for primary prophylaxis due to a high complication rate but is effective in reducing re-bleeding rates, but again does not alter overall mortality.
- Band ligation is as effective as sclerotherapy with a lower complication rate in preventing re-bleeding but again does not alter overall mortality.
- Alcoholic cirrhosis accounts for 20% of European liver transplants. A 6-month period of abstinence prior to transplantation is usually required; some patients recover sufficiently during this period.

This patient has severe hyponatraemia but he also has oedema and ascites and therefore a higher then normal body sodium concentration, but an even greater excess of water.

Hyponatraemia occurs as a result of a number of factors:
- Hypoalbuminaemia reduces the plasma colloid osmotic pressure, reducing return of water from the interstitial compartment to the intravascular compartment and therefore contributing to the ascites and hyponatraemia.
- Reduced intravascular volume results in low renal blood flow, a prerenal uraemia and stimulation of renin and aldosterone release. Aldosterone stimulates the reabsorption of sodium from the distal renal tubules.
- Intravascular volume depletion stimulates ADH secretion directly with enhanced free water reabsorption also causing a dilutional hyponatraemia.

a) 3. Involvement of eye movements.

4. Sensory changes on nerve conduction studies.

b) 1. Riluzole.

Amyotrophic lateral sclerosis is one form of motor neuron disease (MND). Progressive motor weakness and bulbar dysfunction lead to premature death, usually from respiratory failure. Patients often have a combination of upper and lower motor signs in the same limb. Oculomotor involvement is not seen.

MRI abnormalities due to corticospinal tract degeneration do occur in MND. A raised CK (>1000) is unusual but can occur with rapid de-innervation. Electrophysiological tests are confirmatory but not diagnostic. In typical MND, nerve conduction velocity is normal (slow conduction suggests a demyelinating neuropathy), sensory studies are normal and electromyography reveals diffuse fibrillation and fasiculation. Sensory abnormalities on NCS should lead to the diagnosis being questioned. Dementia occurs in 3% of patients with ALS. In typical ALS a lumbar puncture is often normal but a moderately raised protein level can be found.

A lumbar puncture may help exclude treatable conditions, for example:
1. In pure upper motor neuron syndromes (spastic paraparesis) to exclude primary progressive mutiple sclerosis
2. If a paraprotein is present on serum electrophoresis to help exclude an underlying paraneoplastic process
3. In young patients where, with rapidly progressive disease, there are remote possibilities such as poisoning, immunologically-mediated neuropathies or porphoria.

Riluzole is a glutamate antagonist and is licensed for the treatment of MND. Clinical trials have shown a variable benefit of between 3 and 6 months prolongation of pre-tracheostomy survival.

The other treatments listed have not been shown to have a consistent benefit on survival outcomes.

1. **An echocardiogram may show abrupt displacement of both mitral valve leaflets.**

The signs are consistent with mitral valve prolapse; this can place excessive pressure on the papillary muscles and lead to myocardial ischaemia and chest pain. This often does not bare any relation to exercise and exercise testing is often negative.

Prolapse of the mitral valve is a common condition and the majority of cases are idiopathic and the majority of patients are asymptomatic.

It may be associated with rheumatic and ischaemic heart disease and is also associated with Marfan's syndrome, pseudoxanthoma elasticum, Ehlers–Danlos syndrome and *Osteogenesis imperfecta*.

With standing or during the Valsalva manoeuvre, ventricular volume will get smaller and therefore the sounds will move earlier in systole because the ventricle will fill more quickly.

A minority of patients with mitral valve prolapse develop chest pain which is commonly atypical. It is often associated with inferior T-wave ECG changes.

Ventricular ectopic beats are common with mitral regurgitation. Ventricular arrythmias occur much less often and they are rarely life threatening.

A characteristic echocardigraphic finding is mid-systolic prolapse of the posterior mitral valve leaflet into the left atrium.

The risks of endocarditis warrant prophylactic antibiotics.

Answer to question 120

a) 1. Acute promyelocytic leukaemia.

b) 2. Bone marrow examination.

Acute promyelocytic leukaemia (acute myleloid leukaemia subtype M3) is associated with a high incidence of bleeding at diagnosis due to expression of tissue factor on the leukaemic cells causing disseminated intravascular coagulation. In combination with the raised level of myeloblasts it is therefore the most likely **underlying** diagnosis in this case. The diagnosis is best confirmed with a bone marrow examination. This will reveal characteristic hypergranular blasts.

*Note: a fibrinogen below 1.0 g/L, a platelet count of less then 100×10^9/L and a thrombin time of more than double the control value is considered virtually diagnostic of disseminated intravascular coagulation (DIC).

Disseminated intravascular coagulation occurs as a result of inappropriate and excessive activation of the haemostatic system. The coagulation cascade is activated leading to excessive amounts of thrombin and the formation of fibrin strands; in combination with activated platelets these produce fibrin-platelet plugs which act as a fine mesh sieve – as red cells pass through they are distorted leading to intravascular haemolysis and the production of red cell fragments (schistocytes and helmut cells). The coagulation pathway is then activated and all coagulation factors and fibrin and platelets are consumed. Liver and marrow synthesis is unable to keep up with demand.

The major clinical manifestation is usually bleeding. This can vary from mild to severe and runs an acute or chronic course. Bleeding can present as:

- Haematomas, often over pressure-dependent areas
- Around venepuncture sites around indwelling lines
- More generalized haemorrhage throughout the gastrointestinal tract and other organ systems
- 5–10% present with microthrombotic lesions leading to gangrene of the fingers or toes.

The management of DIC is difficult and requires a multidisciplinary approach:

1. Treat the underlying cause: broad-spectrum antibiotics should be given in all cases. In obstetric emergencies complete evacuation of the uterus can be life-saving.
2. Acute bleeding with shock requires fluid resuscitation.
3. Bleeding requires supportive therapy with FFP and platelets.
4. Experimental treatments include the use of activated protein C and low molecular weight heparin.

Summary of expected haematological and biochemical changes in DIC

Hb	↓
Platelets	↓
PT	↑
APPT	↑
Fibrinogen	↓
FDP	↑
Schistocytes/helmut cells (fragmented red cells)	↑
Unconjugated bilirubin	↑
LDH	↑

Causes of disseminated intravascular coagulation:

Infections
- Septicaemia (accounts for 60% of cases); usually gram-negative bacteria
- Viraemia
- Protozoa (malaria)

Malignancy
- Metastatic Ca
- Acute promyelocytic leukaemias

Obstetric disorders
- Septic abortion
- Abruptio placentae
- Eclampsia
- Amniotic fluid embolism

Shock
- Surgical trauma
- Burns
- Heat stroke

Liver disease
- Cirrhosis

Other causes
- Cardiac bypass surgery
- Transplantation
- ABO incompatible transfusion
- Snake bites
- Acute pancreatitis
- Accelerated phase hypertension
- Methaemoglobinaemia

4. Renal cell carcinoma.

- The chronic history of anorexia, weight loss and fever raise the broad differential of sepsis or malignancy.
- The combination of polycythaemia, hypercalcaemia and blood on urinalysis is best explained by a hypernephroma.
- The most likely bronchial malignancy that would cause hypercalcaemia would be a squamous cell carcinoma but this does not readily explain the haemoglobin level or the haematuria.
- Haematuria is present in 50% of patients with hypernephroma.
- The classical triad of haematuria, flank pain and a flank mass occurs in only 10–20% of patients.
- Hypernephromas are a well-recognized malignancy to present atypically, e.g. with steroid-resistant polymyalgic symptoms.
- Radical nephrectomy is the treatment of choice.

b) 2. Atrial fibrillation with pre-excitation.

d) 4. IV flecainide.

The rapid irregular ventricular rates and the absence of any cardiovascular risk factors mean that the diagnosis is most likely to be atrial fibrillation with pre-excitation (conduction via an accessory pathway). This is most likely to be due to the Wolff-Parkinson-White syndrome.

In this case the patient appears to be haemodynamically stable. Chemical cardioversion should therefore be attempted and IV flecainide would be the most appropriate drug. Flecainide is a Vaughn Williams class IC drug that results in sodium channel blockade and slowing of conduction in all cardiac cells including the anomalous pathways responsible for the Wolff-Parkinson-White syndrome.

Verapamil is contraindicated because it blocks conduction via the atrioventricular node and enhances conduction via the accessory pathway, which can increase the ventricular rate further.

If episodes are frequent and symptomatic then the definitive treatment is radiofrequency ablation. This may prevent the occurrence of atrial fibrillation but more importantly it prevents the possibility of degeneration into ventricular fibrillation. Normally in atrial fibrillation, ventricular depolarization is prevented by the gating effect of the atrioventricular node. In patients with an accessory pathway and a short refractory period this can be lost, with progression to ventricular fibrillation.

1. Methaemoglobinaemia.

From the shape of the oxygen dissociation curve, one would predict an oxygen saturation of 98% with a PaO_2 of 110 mmHg. The explanation for a low saturation with a normal–high PaO_2 is that something has decreased the ability of haemoglobin to bind oxygen. Both carboxyhaemoglobin and methaemoglobin can do this. Note that pulse oximetry cannot distinguish between oxyhaemoglobin, carboxyhaemoglobin and methaemoglobin because they use only two wavelengths of light. Blood gas analysers will give a true record of the saturation.

Methaemoglobinaemia causes a variable degree of cyanosis and should be considered in any patient with significant central cyanosis in whom there is no evidence of cardiorespiratory disease. The degree of cyanosis produced by 5 g/dL of deoxygenated haemoglobin can be produced by 1.5 g/dL of methaemoglobin. Methaemoglobin levels of 10–20% can be tolerated well in patients with lifelong disease but individuals who have accumulated a similar level acutely after exposure to drugs or toxins may be acutely dyspnoeic.

Methaemoglobulinaemia may arise:

1. *As a result of a genetic defect in red cell metabolism*: *NADH diaphorase deficiency*. NADH diaphorase catalyses a major step in the pathway for haemoglobin reduction. The condition is inherited as autosomal recessive. Homozygotes have elevated levels of methaemoglobin and are cyanosed from birth. Heterozygotes do not have elevated levels of methaemoglobin but are susceptible to the antioxidant actions of drugs such as antimalarial agents. Crises can be treated with ascorbic acid or methylene blue (methylene blue reduces metHb to Hb).
2. *As a genetic defect of haemoglobin structure*. There are several abnormal haemoglobin variants all of which are designated haemoglobin M. Cyanosis is usually present from birth. They are all inherited as autosomal dominant. They will not respond to treatment with ascorbic acid or methylene blue.
3. *Acquired methaemoglobinaemia*. This is usually a result of the administration of drugs or exposure to chemicals that cause oxidation of haemoglobin. Agents include nitrites (commonly used as preservatives), phenacitin, primiquin dapsone, sulphonamides and various aniline dye derivatives. The drug or chemical agent should be discontinued if possible.

a) 5. Right axis deviation.

   6. Right bundle branch block.

b) 3. Osteum secundum atrial septal defect.

The oxygen saturation in the RA and SVC should be the same; however, there is a step up in oxygen saturation at the level of the mid RA. This can only result from the addition of oxygenated blood to the deoxygenated blood in the right heart circulation, i.e. an abnormal connection between the right and left sides of the heart. Since this is occurring in the atria, it must be due to an atrial septal defect (ASD). The location of the step up is suggestive of an osteum secondum defect as this lesion occurs mid-way down in the A–V septum.

Osteum secundum ASDs are also associated with right bundle branch block and right axis deviation; whereas right bundle branch block and left axis deviation is associated with ostium primum ASDs.

Atrial septal defects are the second commonest cause of congenital cardiac disease in adults after bicuspid aortic valves. They most commonly present as:
- Incidental findings
- Atrial arrhythmias
- Exertional fatigue or dyspnoea
- Right heart failure
- Paradoxical embolism/cerebral abscess.

Increased flow through the pulmonary circulation will elevate pulmonary artery pressure and eventually lead to reversal of the left-to-right shunt – Eisenmenger's syndrome.

a) 3. Gout.

b) 1. Start oral prednisolone.

The patient presents with severe polyarticular gout. The visualization of negatively birefringent crystals indicating monosodium urate monohydrate deposition in the joints is pathognomic of gout.

Gout arises due to the deposition of monosodium urate crystals in tissue. This most commonly leads to:
  1. An acute inflammatory arthritis
  2. Tophus formation
  3. Nephrolithiasis and urolithiasis
  4. Chronic renal disease and hypertension
  5. Chronic erosive changes and a deforming arthritis.

Acute gout typically presents with a hot, red, swollen, tender joint. The first metatarsophalangeal joint is commonly involved at presentation. Other joints involved include the ankle, knee and tarsal area. The most significant differential to exclude is sepsis. Simple analgesics and NSAIDS can ease pain. All NSAIDs should be avoided in this patient with impaired renal function, anaemia and a previous history of suspected coffee ground vomit.

Colchicine is often the first line treatment for acute gout in the context of renal failure but should be prescribed at a reduced dose. Common side-effects include abdominal pain and diarrhoea. Colchicine 500 mcg bd has not been effective in this patient; increasing the dose is unlikely to work and carries the risk of increased toxicity, particularly in a patient with background myelosuppression. Having confirmed the diagnosis of gout, and in the absence of sepsis, corticosteroids represent the best management option.

3. Rescue angioplasty.

The ECG changes present here indicate that the patient has sustained an **inferior myocardial infarction.** Infarction in this area often leads to **bradycardia** because the right coronary artery, which supplies this territory, also supplies the junctional tissues.

Given that the patient's blood pressure is still maintained and he is still conscious the first treatment that should be given is IV atropine. This is an antimuscarinic agent that blocks vagal tone.

The presence of continued chest pain and unresolved ECG segments is an indication that clot lysis has not been achieved. Rescue angioplasty is the treatment of choice in cases where there is evidence that reperfusion has not been achieved with fibrinolytic treatment.

All randomized controlled clinical trials of **primary angioplasty** have shown a reduced incidence of stroke, recurrent ischaemia and the need for new target vessel revascularization compared to thrombolysis.

It should be noted, however, that such results were achieved in specific centres working under trial conditions.

a) 4. Atherosclerotic renal artery stenosis.

b) 1. Renal ultrasound.

Atheromatous renal artery stenosis is the likely diagnosis in this patient with vascular disease, hypertension, impaired renal function and intermittent episodes of pulmonary oedema. Bilateral renal artery stenosis is a well-recognized cause of recurrent pulmonary oedema. Explanations for the intermittent episodes of pulmonary oedema include hypertensive increased afterload, inability of the hypertrophied left ventricle to relax in diastole and sodium retention due to activation of the renin-angiotensin system.

The degree of left ventricular impairment would be unlikely to account for the severity and frequency of presentation in this patient. The aortic valve gradient in the presence of preserved left ventricular function would also be unlikely to result in such a presentation with rapid recovery. It is, however, important to realize that impaired left ventricular function can lead to underestimation of the gradient across the aortic valve determined by ECHO.

After obesity and chronic alcohol abuse, renal artery stenosis is the commonest secondary cause of hypertension. It is commoner in whites than blacks. Other clues that it may be the underlying diagnosis in a hypertensive patient include a deterioration in renal function after commencing an ACEI or angiotensin II receptor blocker, an abdominal unilateral systolic-diastolic bruit (low sensitivity but high specificity) and a unilateral small kidney detected at ultrasound.

The two main causes of renal artery stenosis are (i) atheromatous disease which is commoner in elderly males and affects the proximal part of the renal artery and (ii) fibromuscular hyperplasia which occurs in young females and affects either the distal main renal artery or the intrarenal portion.

Renal ultrasound with duplex sonograhy in experienced hands is an effective initial screening method for renal artery stenosis. Digital subtraction angiography remains the gold standard investigation. Other less invasive tests include MR angiography, spiral CT angiography and captopril renography.

Correctable therapy is either percutaneous transluminal renal angioplasty with or without stenting or surgical revascularization, together with modifiable risk factors. Some elderly patients may be treated medically with a combination of ACEI and diuretics. Elevated cholesterol levels should be aggressively treated.

a) 4. Glucagonoma.

b) 2. Raised fasting glucagon levels.

Glucagonomas are alpha-cell pancreatic tumours that secrete glucagon and other related pancreatic peptides. They are present in adult life and are more common in females than males. Patients typically present with a necrolytic migratory rash and diabetes mellitus; other features include weight loss, diarrhoea and venous thrombosis.

The diagnosis is confirmed by finding elevated fasting plasma glucagon levels.

Surgical excision is the treatment of choice, and if removal is complete, it is associated with complete resolution of symptoms. Many of these tumours are, however, widely disseminated at the time of diagnosis. Streptozotocin may be used to reduce metastasis size and symptoms; arterial embolization may be used to treat hepatic secondaries. The diabetes is usually insulin-dependent, anticoagulation will reduce the risk of thrombosis and oral zinc supplements may help the rash.

5. Chronic myeloid leukaemia.

The most likely diagnosis is **chronic myeloid leukaemia** (also termed chronic granulocytic leukaemia). This is a clonal disease that results from an acquired genetic change in a pleuripotential stem cell.

Symptoms include lethargy, weight loss and haemorrhage. Increased sweating is characteristic. Fever and lymphadenopathy are rare in the chronic phase.

Pain or discomfort in the splenic area is typical and splenic infarction can lead to severe episodes of pain. Visual disturbances can occur and these are due to retinal haemorrhages. 60–80% of patients have splenomegaly at the time of diagnosis; the liver is also often enlarged. Ecchymosis may be present (these are raised areas of subcutaneous bleeding). Patients who present with splenomegaly are usually anaemic.

The leucocyte concentration is between 50 and 200×10^9/L. A neutrophilia is characteristic. The percentage of eosinophils and basophils are also increased (absence of a basophilia casts doubt on the diagnosis). Platelet numbers are increased to the range of $300–600 \times 10^9$/L. The blood film typically shows a full range of cells in the granulocyte series. The neutrophil alkaline phosphatase score is **low** in chronic myeloid leukaemia in 95% of cases (this contrasts with myelodysplasia where the NAP score is typically high).

The diagnosis is confirmed by chromosomal analysis to confirm the 9:22 translocation – the Philadelphia chromosome. A bone marrow examination is best used to perform cytogenetic analysis.

Other notes
- **Myelodysplasia.** The myelodysplastic syndromes are a morphological heterogeneous group of conditions where haematopoetic cells show abnormalities in proliferation and maturation. They have a tendency to evolve into acute leukaemia.
  - The majority of patients are **elderly.**
  - Patients present with bone marrow failure – with symptoms of anaemia (either normocytic or macrocytic), sepsis and bleeding due to pancytopenia.
  - Splenomegaly is present in 10% of patients.
  - 20% have anaemia in combination with neutropenia or thrombocytopenia.
  - If there is a leucocytosis then it is usually a monocytosis, sometimes with a neutrophilia. The findings of an increased number of **eosinophils or basophils is very uncommon.**
  - The neutrophil alkaline phosphatase score will be **normal or raised.**

- A **leukaemoid reaction** is a reactive and excessive leucocytosis usually characterized by the presence of immature white cells as well as mature white cells in the peripheral blood. They are usually seen in association with infection, and occasionally with severe haemolysis or metastatic cancer. Associated granulocyte changes include toxic granulation, Dohle bodies and a high neutrophil alkaline phosphatase score.

Immature white cells (left shift) and nucleated red blood cells in the peripheral blood constitutes a leucoerythroblastic blood film:

Causes of a leuco-erythroblastic blood film

Bone marrow infiltration
- Carcinoma, lymphoma, chronic myeloid leukaemia, multiple myeloma, Gauchers disease

Myeloproliferative disorders
- Acute myeloid leukaemia and the myelodysplastic syndromes
- Idiopathic myelofibrosis
- Chronic myeloid leukaemia

Infections
- Tuberculosis, Severe sepsis

Haemoglobinopathies
- Sickle cell crises, thalassemia

Shock
- Severe haemorrhage

Other
- Systemic lupus erythematosus
- Nutritional disorders
- Severe megaloblastic anaemia

a) 5. Adrenal failure secondary to tuberculosis.

b) 1. Hydrocortisone and fludrocortisone.

The biochemical picture of hyponatraemia, hyperkalaemia, a moderately increased urea, and hypoglycaemia is typical. Moderate corrected hypercalcaemia is also a recognized feature of adrenal failure. Glucocorticoid replacement, typically hydrocortisone 20-30mg a day in divided doses. Mineralocorticoid replacement with fludrocortisone 0.1 mg o.d. may be necessary.

Note:
- The low T4 raises the possibility of secondary adrenal failure but the increased TSH indicates normal pituitary function. A low T4 and high TSH are frequently seen in Addison's disease in the absence of functional hypothyroidism, and revert to normal following steroid replacement.
- Addison's disease in the western world is most commonly autoimmune in nature and is associated with autoimmune hypothyroidism in approximately 10% of cases. In this case, the absence of thyroid antibodies and the patient's race puts tuberculosis higher on the list of causes of adrenal failure.

The diagnosis may be confirmed by:
1. The short synacthen test – 250 mcg of tetracosactrin is administered, followed by measurement of cortisol levels at 0, 30 and 60 min. Failure of cortisol to increase by 250 nmol/L at 30 min to a level greater than 550 nmol/L confirms the diagnosis.
2. Measurement of ACTH levels – elevated in primary adrenal failure.
3. Abdominal X-ray – evidence of adrenal calcification with tuberculous adrenal destruction.
4. Measurement of adrenal autoantibodies.

5. Trifascicular block.

This is the combination of 1st degree heart block, left axis deviation and right bundle branch block. Combined with symptoms suggestive of syncope this would be an indication for a permanent pacemaker.

1st degree block (PR >5 small squares 0.2 s)

This indicates that conduction through the atrioventricular node has been delayed.

Causes of 1st degree block:
- Normal variant
- Ischaemic heart disease
- Hypokalaemia
- Drugs – digoxin, quinidine, beta blockers, diltiazem

Other causes:
- Lyme disease
- Acute rheumatic endocarditis.

Right bundle branch block

The QRS complex is broad (>3 small squares) and there is an R wave in V1 and a small Q wave in V6 (caused by septal depolarization from left to right).

The causes of right bundle branch block are:
- Ischaemic heart disease
- Cardiomyopathy
- Atrial septal defect
- Ebstein's anomaly*
- Massive pulmonary embolism.

*Ebstein's anomaly is a congenital defect of the tricuspid valve leading to tricuspid regurgitation. In the majority of cases it is associated with an ASD.

The ECG axis

In the majority of cases the axis can be calculated very quickly as follows:
- A positive QRS complex in leads I and II indicates that the axis is normal.
- If the QRS complex in lead I is positive this effectively rules out right axis deviation.
- If lead II is then negative this indicates that left axis deviation is present.
- A predominantly negative complex in lead I and a positive complex in lead II indicates that right axis deviation is most likely to be present.

Causes of left axis deviation:
- Left anterior hemiblock – can occur as a result of fibrosis or infarction of the conducting system.
- Wolff-Parkinson-White syndrome
- Inferior myocardial infarction
- Ventricular tachycardia
- Left ventricular hypertrophy – (due to fibrosis of the left ventricle leading to left anterior hemiblock).
- Hyperkalaemia
- Tricuspid atresia
- Osteum primum atrial septal defect.

Right axis deviation occurs when the mean frontal axis is >90. It can be a normal finding but more often indicates:
- Right ventricular hypertrophy
- Wolff-Parkinson-White syndrome
- Antereolateral myocardial infarction
- Dextrocardia
- Left posterior hemiblock.

> **5.** Arrange for PEG insertion with consent in her best interests by her nominated consultant.

This patient, who has a receptive and expressive dysphasia, is unlikely to have the capacity to understand and give consent.

There are three stages of capacity:
  1. Comprehension and retention of information
  2. Ability to believe information
  3. Ability to weigh information and make a decision.

Other members of the family or next of kin cannot give consent (consent by proxy) under English law.

Clearly PEG insertion would not take place without a fully informed discussion with the family and other members of the healthcare team.

Other notes
- Parenteral nutrition, i.e. nutrition directly into the blood stream, should only be used in patients with intestinal failure who are unable to meet their nutritional needs via the gastrointestinal tract.
- Post-operative and intensive care patients are the largest group of patients who require short-term parental feeding.
- While in practice there may be some repeated attempts at a nasogastric tube insertion, a clearly defined plan needs to be made regarding future nutritional support in a patient who is unlikely to regain her swallowing reflex in the immediate short term.

a) 2. Guillain–Barré syndrome (acute inflammatory demyelinating polyneuropathy).

b) 1. IV immunoglobulin.

2. Sedation and intubation.

The Guillain–Barré syndrome (GBS) (also known as acute inflammatory demyelinating polyneuropathy (AIDP)) is typically characterized by a polyneuropathy that develops over the course of a few days up to a maximum of 4 weeks.

* Note: this patient is developing incipient respiratory failure due to a progressive decline in respiratory muscle function. Patients with GBS are at risk of this and they are therefore closely observed, with serial spirometry patients with FVC <20 mL/kg likely to require ventilation. She is therefore going to require **sedation and intubation**.

Symptoms are most commonly preceded by an infection. Respiratory infection is the commonest infection. Twenty percent have gastroenteritis. *Campylobactor jejunii* is the most commonly identified pathogen. These cases are associated with slower recovery, more residual disability and axonal degeneration. GBS has also been associated with other infections such as cytomegalovirus and HIV. The commonest initial symptom in GBS is limb weakness, which is more distal then proximal. A facial nerve palsy is present in 50%, and less frequently, bulbar weakness, opthalmoplegia and tongue weakness is present. In severe cases the respiratory muscles are affected. Eighty percent have sensory symptoms; pain is the commonest symptom and it is usually severe. Autonomic dysfunction is seen in two-thirds (this patient has postural hypotension). Progressive motor weakness and areflexia are therefore the prime requirements for diagnosis.

Investigation

- In the cerebrospinal fluid an elevated protein level and, in particular, a rising protein on serial samples with 10 or fewer mononuclear cells strongly supports the diagnosis. (The presence of more then 50 mononuclear cells should raise doubt about the diagnosis. HIV is particularly associated with a pleocytosis).
- MR imaging can be used but is not specific; it can be useful though to rule out other conditions. Gadolinium enhancement is a non-specific feature that is seen in inflammatory conditions and is caused by disruption of the blood nerve barrier.
- The characteristic electrophysiological changes seen in AIDP (the commonest variant of GBS) reflects segmental demyelination (conduction velocities are decreased and F waves are prolonged or absent).
- Gangliosides are important surface molecules in the nervous system. Antibodies formed against ganglioside epitopes on the surface C jejuni

cross-react with peripheral nerves causing damage. Antiganglioside antibodies are therefore associated with variants of GBS.

Treatment

- Corticosteroids have not been shown to have any consistent beneficial effects.
- Intravenous immunoglobulin may act through anti-idiotypic suppression of autoantibodies and, when started within 2 weeks, seems to have as much effect as plasma exchange and fewer contraindications. It is therefore the initial treatment of choice. Relapses have been noted and it is possible to give another treatment cycle. The main side-effects are myalgias, fevers and chills. An aseptic meningitis can develop and anaphylactic reactions are reported.
- Plasma exchange started in the first 2 weeks of the illness can reduce the length of hospital stay, the duration of mechanical ventilation and the time to reach ambulation. Associated complications are: hypotension, septicaemia, hypocalcaemia and abnormal clotting. Treatment is therefore reserved for severe cases who may not be responding to immunoglobulin treatment.
- The overall outcome for GBS is good with two-thirds making a complete recovery. Ventilatory support is required in 25% of patients.

Other notes

- Acute inflammatory demyelinating polyneuropathy is the commonest variant of GBS but other patterns are described such as acute motor axonal neuropathy, acute motor sensory axonal neuropathy, and the Millar-Fisher syndrome which consists of a triad of ataxia, areflexia and opthalmoplegia. It may also be associated with mild limb weakness, ptosis, and facial and bulbar palsy. It accounts for 5% of patients with GBS.
- *Lyme borreliosis* is a multisystem disease caused by a tick-borne spirochaete, *Borrelia burgdorferi* and acute infection can be associated with cranial neuropathies or radiculopathies.

2. Cryoglobulinaemia.

Her presentation is most consistent with cryoglobulinaema.
- A markedly low C4 occurs in 90% of patients with cryoglobulinaemia.
- Other conditions that may be associated with a low C4: systemic lupus erythematosus (usually low C3, C4), hereditary angioedema.

Conditions where Raynaud's phenomenon may be exhibited
- Systemic lupus erythematosus
- Scleroderma
- Rheumatiod arthritis
- Trauma
- Leukaemia
- Arteriosclerosis
- Mixed cryoglobulinaemia
- Monoclonal gammopathies
- Cold agglutinins

Cryoglobulinaemia occurs as a result of an immune complex mediated vasculitis and vascular obstruction by cryoglobulins. Cryoglobulins are immunoglobulins that precipitate irreversibly in the cold, usually at 4°C.

In the majority of patients with cryoglobulinaemia, an underlying condition in the form of malignant paraproteinaemias, lymphomas, autoimmune diseases or infections is evident.

There are three types of cryoglobulinaemia:
- Type I – the cryoprecipitate is composed of a single monoclonal immunoglobulin without any antibody activity. This can be found in patients with multiple myeloma, Waldenstrom's macroglobinaemia or idiopathic monoclonal gammopathy.
- Type II – usually monoclonal immunoglobulin IgM to polyclonal IgG (rheumatoid factors). Many cases were initially labelled as essential cryoglobulinaemia because no underlying cause could be found. It has now been found that many of these patients have underlying hepatitis C infection.
- Type III – polyclonal IgM and polyclonal IgG.

Mixed cryoglobulinaemias account for most cryoglobulinaemias (60–70%). Other causes of type II and III cryoglobulinaemia include connective tissue diseases, leukaemia, hepatobiliary diseases, infectious diseases and post-infectious glomeronephritis.

Type I cryoglobulins may occur in either sex and are characterized by features of hyperviscosity and vasculitis. These include Raynaud's phenomenon, arterial thrombosis, gangrene and retinal haemorrhage.

Mixed cryoglobulins affect females in particular and present most commonly with a triad of skin, renal and joint disease:

Skin

Cutaneous vasculitis is seen in virtually all patients with prominent lower limb purpura, often progressing to frank ulceration.

Renal

Renal disease due to membranoproliferative glomerulonephritis with immunoglobulin and complement deposition occurs in up to 50% of all patients with mixed cryoglobulinaemia and almost exclusively with type II cryoglobulinaemia. Nephrotic syndrome and hypertension are common sequelae.

Joints

Symmetrical arthralgia affecting the hands, knees and elbows is common in mixed cryoglobulinaemia but rarely progresses to frank arthritis.

Other notes
Common causes of renal impairment associated with a low C3:
- Systemic lupus erythamatosus – C4 usually low
- Idiopathic mesangiocapillary glomerulonephritis type II (type II is associated with facial lipodystrophy) – C4 normal as C3 nephritic factor Ab activates alternative pathway
- Post-streptococcal nephritis – C4 often low
- Infective endocarditis – C4 often low
- Shunt nephritis – C4 often low.

a) 3. Ventricular septal rupture.

b) 2. Immediate consideration for surgery.

When ventricular rupture complicates myocardial infarction the mortality is high. Reperfusion therapy has reduced the incidence from 1–3% to under 1%.

Septal rupture occurs more frequently with anterior then other types of myocardial infarction.

Septal rupture results in a left-to-right shunt with right ventricular overload, increased pulmonary blood flow and secondary overload of the left atrium and ventricle.

As left ventricular systolic function deteriorates and forward flow declines, compensatory vasoconstriction leads to increased systemic vascular resistance; this increases further the size of the shunt.

Typically the time of onset is 24 h or less for those who have received thrombolysis, and is longer without reperfusion.

Clinical manifestations of septal rupture include chest pain, shortness of breath and evidence of low cardiac output and shock. There is a harsh pan systolic murmur along the left sternal border, radiating to the base apex and the right parasternal area. As cardiac shock progresses, these signs may be difficult to detect because the volume of the shunt will start to decrease.

Characteristics of ventricular septal rupture, rupture of the ventricular free wall and papillary muscle rupture			
	Ventricular septal rupture	Rupture of the ventricular free wall	Papillary muscle rupture
Features	Harsh pansystolic murmur thrill, accentuated second sound, gallop rhythm, cardiogenic shock. Left-to-right shunt on colour flow Doppler echocardiography trough the ventricular septum	JVP↑, pulsus paradoxus, electromechanical dissociation, cardiogenic shock Echo-sensitive for effusions >5 mm	A soft murmur, variable signs of RV overload, severe pulmonary oedema, hypotension

Compared to acute mitral regurgitation, septal rupture has a loud murmur, a thrill and right ventricular failure but is less often characterized by severe pulmonary oedema.

'Pump failure' post-myocardial infarction can either be due to significant mechanical complications such as ventricular septal rupture or free wall rupture. It may also be caused by infarction or ischaemia of a large area, ischaemic mitral regurgitation, right ventricular dysfunction or hypovolaemia. Doppler echocardiography is the investigation of choice.

Treatment consists of mechanical support with an intraaortic ballon pump, afterload reduction and ionotropic agents. Early surgical closure is of greatest benefit regardless of clinical state, which contradicts the long-held view that the myocardium was too fragile for early surgical repair.

6. Send dermal punch biopsies for collagen biochemical analysis.

From the family history given it would not be possible to determine the genetic pattern in this family. Typical inheritance is AD.

- Bone mineral densitrometry T scores compare bone density to peak bone mass, therefore this may not be used in a child who has yet to obtain peak bone mass.
- Z scores compare density to age-matched controls and these would be difficult to find for children of this age group. Bone mineral densitometry is highly likely to be abnormal if the patient has osteogenesis imperfecta (OI).
- Routine biochemical indices are normal in patients with OI.
- Collagen biochemistry and genetic linkage analysis are considered the 'Gold Standard' investigation, however, these remain insensitive. Genetic linkage analysis also requires a clear family history and division into affected and unaffected family members, which is not available in this case.

Osteogenesis imperfecta is the commonest inherited disorder of bone. It is characterized by a collagen defect that results in a clinical spectrum ranging from mild forms with few fractures and normal mobility to a severe lethal form with multiple intrauterine fractures and death in the perinatal period. OI has been classified into four types: I, II, II and IV.

Type I is the most frequent and least serious form, and accounts for 60% of all patients with the disorder. Fractures can be delayed until the early perimenopause. After the menopause the fracture rate can be up to seven times normal. The vertebral bone mineral content can be 70% of normal.

Blueness of the sclerae is a particularly important physical sign of OI and, combined with an appropriate history, is virtually diagnostic.

The cardiac manifestations of OI are also important: aortic incompetence, aortic root widening and mitral valve prolapse all occur. Patients with OI often show hypermobility of joints, with resultant flat feet, hyperextensible large joints and dislocation.

Childhood fractures in type I OI may be numerous, but rarely lead to deformity unless treated inappropriately. Any type of fracture can occur; they become less frequent with age. Overall, fractures are more frequent in the lower limbs. Significant scoliosis is rare. The teeth are often discoloured and the enamel (which is normal) fractures easily from the dentine, leading to rapid erosion of both the first and second dentition.

Type II is nearly always lethal: some children may be born dismembered; whereas others may (rarely) survive the perinatal period, and if they do, the condition merges into the type III form.

a) 1. Middle and anterior cerebral artery territory.

b) 2. Carotid doppler of neck vessels.

Infarction of one cerebral hemisphere may cause contralateral hemiparesis or hemiplegia, hemisensory loss or homonymous hemianopia.

- A large cortical stroke in the middle or middle and anterior cerebral artery territories (sometimes termed a total anterior circulation syndrome (TACS)) is recognized by a combination of weakness with or without sensory deficit of two out of three body areas (arm, leg and face) plus a homonymous hemianopia plus new higher cerebral dysfunction (e.g. dysphasia or apraxia).
- A cortical stroke in a branch of the middle or anterior cerebral territories may present with any two of higher cerebral dysfunction, visual field defect and limb weakness or just higher cerebral dysfunction or any restricted motor/sensory defect (such as hand weakness). This is sometimes termed a partial anterior circulation syndrome (PACS).
- A lacunar infarction is due to a small infarct in the basal ganglia, thalamus, internal capsule, cerebral peduncle and pons. Higher cortical function is normal and the patient is conscious. Their presentation may be characteristic:

Pure motor stroke

This is complete or incomplete weakness of one side of the body, involving the whole of two out of the three body areas (face, upper limb or leg). Sensory symptoms, but not signs, may be present and there may be dysarthria and sometimes dysphagia.

Pure sensory stroke

In sensory stroke, there are symptoms and/or sensory signs (but not impaired joint position sense alone) in the same distribution as pure motor stroke.

Sensory motor stroke

This is a combination of pure motor and pure sensory stroke, but without any other features.

Ataxic hemiparesis

Ataxic hemiparesis is a combination of hemiparesis and ipsilateral cerebellar ataxia, often with marked dysarthria, clumsiness of the hand and unsteadiness.

a) 1. EMG.

2. Serum creatinine kinase.

7. MRI scan of the right thigh.

b) 1. Dermatomyositis.

He has a degree of proximal weakness (difficulty with ladders) tender muscles and the classical rash of dermatomyositis (see below).

Dermatomyositis and polymyositis are the commonest forms of an idiopathic inflammatory myopathy. They have an annual incidence of 2–10 cases per million.

- Proximal muscle weakness is the dominating clinical feature in both conditions and is almost universal.
- Myalgia is present in 50% of cases.
- In addition to the characteristic rash, three of the four criteria listed below are required to make the diagnosis of dermatomyositis.
- The clinical presentation may overlap with other autoimmune rheumatic diseases.
- An underlying malignancy is present in up to 15% of patients with dermatomyositis and 10% of patients with polymyositis. The highest risk appears to be in patients over 45 years old who lack characteristic autoantibodies, or in patients who have overlap/undifferentiated autoimmune rheumatic disease.
- Specific investigations should therefore be broadened and include a chest X-ray, urinalysis and faecal occult blood testing. A prostate-specific antigen level check should be carried out in males, and mammography, pelvic ultrasound and CA125 levels in females.

Criteria for the diagnosis of dermatomyositis/polymyositis (3 of 4 required)
1. Compatable weakness: symmetrical proximal muscle weakness developing over weeks or months
2. Elevated serum muscle enzymes (up to a 50-fold elevation)
3. Characteristic electromyographic findings: myopathic potentials (low amplitude, short duration, polyphasic), fibrillation, complex repetitive discharges
4. Typical muscle biopsy findings

Dermatological features of dermatomyositis:
1. Gottren's papules: purple, flat or raised lesions over the knuckles, elbows, knees and medial malleoli
2. Heliotrope sign: purple rash around the eyes
3. Erythematous and/or poikilodermatous rash – the shawl sign or V sign
4. Mechanic's hands – cracking and fissuring of skin over the finger pads

Other points:

- MRI scanning of the muscle may be helpful in identifying inflamed muscle and can direct the muscle biopsy.
- The CK level is elevated in almost all cases.
- 80–90% of patients have characteristic EMG findings.
- 40–80% of patients with PM and DM are ANA positive.
- Specific antibodies include anti Jo-1, PL-7, PL-12, anti-SRP and anti-Mi 2.
- Myositis associated antibodies also include:
  - Anti RNP – MCTD overlap syndromes
  - Anti PM-Scl – PM-scleroderma overlap
  - Anti Ku – PM-scleroderma overlap.
- Treatments for dermatomyositis include:
  1. Corticosteroids
  2. Methotrexate and azathioprine
  3. IV immunoglobulin.

5. Ventricular tachycardia.

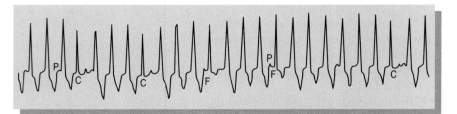

The ECG demonstrates:
- A broad complex tachycardia
- Atrioventricular dissociation (P waves (P) bearing no relationship to the QRS complex)
- Fusion beats (F)
- Capture beats (C)
- Wide and bizarre complexes.

The rhythm is therefore most likely to be ventricular tachycardia.

The presence of wide and bizarre complexes support the diagnosis but only indicate that conduction through the ventricle is abnormal – similar complexes can occur in supraventricular tachycardia with abherrent conduction, or conduction over accessory pathways.

P waves are seen but have no relationship to the QRS complex. It can be difficult to decide whether the P wave is conducted anteriogredely (supraventricular tachycardia (SVT)) or retrogradely (ventricular tachycardia (VT)). If there is atrioventricular dissociation in conjunction with a broad complex tachycardia this is most likely to be ventricular in origin.

Capture beats are narrow QRS complexes followed by an upright T wave. A capture beat is produced by momentary activation of the ventricle by the sinus impulse during AV dissociation.

Fusion beats have morphology between that of a complex produced by an ectopic beat and the QRS of a sinus beat followed by an inverted T wave. Fusion beats indicate that the ventricle has been activated from two foci, with one being ventricular in origin. Both then invade the ventricle simultaneously.

*Note: fusion beats and capture beats are not often seen, but strongly support the diagnosis of ventricular tachycardia.

Other features more commonly seen and also supportive of a diagnosis of VT:
- Ventricular rate >120 (usually between 150–250/min
- QRS duration >0.14 (3.5 small squares)
- Concordance (same QRS direction) in leads V1–V6
- Extreme left or right axis deviation
- Adenosine has no effect but left or right axis deviation may become clearer.

2. Alendronate plus calcium and vitamin D.

Most patients with polymyalgia rheumatica require treatment with steroids for 1–2 years and all patients are older than 50 years.

Bone loss during corticosteroid treatment is mediated by inhibition of gonadal and adrenal steroid production leading to hypogonadism and a direct negative effect on calcium absorption and osteoblast function. Corticosteroid treatment doubles the risk of hip fractures and quadruples the risk of vertebral fractures.

The combination of a once weekly biphosphonate such as alendronate or risedronate plus calcium and vitamin D should be started early to prevent accelelerated bone loss with the introduction of prednisolone.

Polymyalgia rheumatica is a clinical syndrome characterized by proximal girdle pain and stiffness. Muscle weakness is not a feature. It is closely related to giant cell arteritis, which is a large vessel vasculitis. Ninety percent of patients are >60 years old and the majority are female. There are no specific serological tests but elevated acute phase markers are typical.

Both giant cell arteritis and polymyalgia rheumatica are exquisitely sensitive to steroids. The dose of steroids in giant cell arteritis is typically 40–60 mg/day. 10–20 mg is often sufficient in polymyalgia rheumatica. The response to treatment can be measured clinically and by monitoring the acute phase markers.

Osteoporosis is characterized by low bone mass and microarchitectural deterioration in bone tissue leading to an increased bone fragility and fracture rate.

Bone mineral densitrometry defines osteoporosis on the basis of bone mineral density compared to population-matched normal values. The WHO uses a T-score value. An individual with a T-score <–2.5 SD at the spine hip or forearm is classified as having osteoporosis. A T-score of –2.5 to –1 SD is classified as osteopenia and >–1 as healthy. The T-score is calculated by taking the difference between a patient's measured bone mass density (BMD) and the mean BMD of healthy adults at peak bone mass matched for ethnicity and gender, and expressing the difference relative to the standard deviation of that population. The T-score therefore indicates the difference between the patient's BMD and the ideal BMD achieved by a young adult.

BMD can also be expressed as Z score units: in this case the patient is compared to age-matched controls. They are not as widely used as T scores. The spine and femur are generally regarded as the most important BMD measurements because they are the sites at which osteoporotic fractures have the most impact on quality of life.

3. Count numbers out aloud.

Myasthenia gravis is the most likely diagnosis and counting numbers would be a good way of testing for fatigueable weakness, which would be characteristic of myasthenia gravis.

Myasthenia gravis is a neuromuscular disorder characterized by fatigable weakness of the skeletal muscles. This is due to a decrease in the number of acetylcholine receptors at neuromuscular junctions due to antibody mediated autoimmune attack. The typical patient is female and aged 50–60 years. The cardinal features are weakness and fatigue. The course is variable and there can be exacerbations and remissions. The cranial muscles and usually the lids and extraoccular muscles are involved early – leading to diplopia and ptosis. The pupils are never affected. In the majority, the weakness becomes more generalized giving a fatigueable proximal limb weakness, but reflexes will be preserved. The diagnosis may be confirmed with the edrophonium test; the test inhibits acetylcholinesterase preventing the breakdown of acetylcholine resulting in increased muscle power. Repetitive nerve stimulation will demonstrate reduction in the amplitude of action potentials. The antiacetylcholine receptor antibody is detectable in the serum of 80% of all myaesthenic patients and their presence is almost diagnostic; a negative test does not exclude the diagnosis.

Answer to question 142

1. Henoch-Schönlein purpura.

Henoch Schönlein purpura is a small vessel vasculitis consisting of purpuric skin lesions characteristically involving the extensor surfaces of the arms, legs and buttocks.

- It is also commonly associated with a non-migratory arthralgia and abdominal manifestations, including pain, vomiting and intestinal bleeding.
- The renal lesion of Henoch Schönlein purpura is essentially identical to an IgA nephropathy – it is therefore the prototype example of a mesangioproliferative glomerulonephritis.
- The disease is most commonly seen in patients under 20 years of age.
- Renal involvement does not always occur initially but its incidence increases in older patients.
- Haematuria and proteinuria are the most common renal presentations; a minority present with a frank nephritic syndrome.

Other notes
- Mixed essential cryoglobulinaemia can present with palpaple purpura on the legs and nephritis but would be more likely in an older patient.
- Without a rash, IgA nephropathy would be the most probable cause of the urinary findings.
- Minimal change nephropathy tends to present in children with a frank nephrotic syndrome.
- Membranous glomerulonephritis also tends to present with a nephrotic syndrome.

a) 1. Alpha-feto protein levels.

    3. Hepatic ultrasound and Doppler studies.

    7. Hepatitis C PCR.

e) 5. Start spironolactone.

The clinical presentation is consistent with chronic hepatitis C causing cirrhosis and ascites.

Hepatitis C is an RNA virus which is transmitted via contaminated blood and other body secretions. The incubation period varies from 2 weeks to 20 weeks. Most patients are asymptomatic and many present with advanced chronic liver disease.

Eighty percent of patients will develop chronic hepatitis and 30% will develop cirrhosis at 30 years. Other disease associations include cryoglobulinaemia, membranoproliferative glomerulonephritis, porphyria cutanea tarda and thyroiditis.

It is important to confirm the diagnosis of hepatitis C with hepatitis C PCR as false positive antibody results can occur. Alpha-feto protein levels should be measured as patients with chronic hepatitis C are at risk of developing hepatocellular carcinomas.

Hepatic ultrasound with Doppler studies will provide initial information about hepatic architecture and help assess whether there is any evidence of portal hypertension or malignancy.

Other secondary investigations that may be considered in this patient include:
● Proceeding to a CT abdomen for more information if diagnostic uncertainty remains
● Arranging a liver biopsy to assess the severity of liver damage attributable to hepatitis C virus and other pathology

Ascites results from the pathological accumulation of fluid in the peritoneal cavity. It is the commonest complication of portal hypertension and indicates a poor prognosis. Abdominal paracentesis and ascitic fluid analysis in combination with the history and physical findings almost always reveals the cause of ascites. It is mandatory to exclude and treat for bacterial peritonitis in patients admitted with hepatic failure. Other general management measures include:
  1. Salt restriction should be recommended.
  2. Diuretics: usually starting with spironolactone (100 mg/day) and adding further loop diuretics if necessary (gynaecomastia associated with spironolactone may require a change to mmiloride).

Answer to question 143 *(continued)*

3. Therapeutic paracentesis may be necessary if there is massive ascites causing discomfort and respiratory embarrassment.

Summary of main causes of ascites

Cirrhosis	80%
Malignancy	10%
Congestive cardiac failure	
Constrictive pericarditis	
Tuberculosis	10%
Pancreatic disease	

Ascitic tap findings

Appearance
Usually straw coloured and clear
(Milky fluid chylous ascites can result from thoracic duct blockage)

Cell count
*Absolute neutrophil count above 250 cells/mm³ is diagnostic of bacterial infection**

Serum ascites gradient (calculated from extracting the ascitic fluid albumin from serum albumin)
SAAG above 11 g/L indicates portal hypertension with >90% accuracy

Culture
Culture in blood culture bottles
*Spontaneous bacterial endocarditis is present in up to 30% of patients admitted with cirrhosis and ascites

Classification of ascites by serum: ascites albumin gradient

Effectively indicating portal hypertension
High gradient (>11 g/L)
- Cirrhosis
- Alcoholic hepatitis
- Cardiac ascites
- Constrictive pericarditis
- Massive liver metastasis
- Fulminent hepatic failure
- Budd Chiari syndrome
- Veno occlusive diseases
- Myxoedema

Low gradient (<11 g/L)
- Tuberculosis peritonitis
- Pancreatic ascites
- Bowel obstruction/infarction
- Biliary ascites
- Nephrotic syndrome
- Post-operative lymphatic leak
- Serositis

2. Benign paraproteinaemia.

The most likely diagnosis is a benign paraproteinaemia (previously known as a monoclonal gammopathy of uncertain significance (MGUS)).

Mechanical back pain and urinary frequency are common symptoms in this age group and are separate entities to the diagnosis of MGUS.

Benign paraproteinaemias can be found in up to 1% of the healthy population (increasing to 3% in those over 70 years). They may also be found in chronic disease states and in patients with liver disease.

The following criterion should be fulfilled:
- A concentration of paraprotein less then 20 g/dL
- Absence of Bence-Jones protein
- Absence of an immune paresis (in this case, the other immunoglobulins are not depressed)
- A normal skeletal survey
- <4% plasma cells in the bone marrow
  (Strictly therefore, in this case, a bone marrow biopsy would be indicated, but in clinical practice, patients are often followed up on a 6-monthly basis if the paraprotein level is low and the remaining immunoglobulin levels remain normal).

In the case of myeloma one may also expect to find:
- A monoclonal band on serum protein electrophoresis and an immune paresis with or without Bence-Jones proteins in the urine (60% of IgG and IgA myelomas produce Bence-Jones proteins).
- An increased proportion – >10% of plasma cells in the bone marrow aspirate (>30% of plasma cells or plasmocytomas indicates a poorer prognosis).
- X-ray changes showing punched out radiolucent areas in the skull, vertebrae, ribs and pelvis. The alkaline phosphatase level will be normal unless there are fractures or liver involvement.

Criteria for diagnosing myeloma

Major
- Plasmacytoma on biopsy
- >30% of plasma cells on bone marrow biopsy
- Monoclonal band on electrophoresis >35g/L for IgG, 20g/L IgA, or >1.0 g of light chains excreted in the urine per day

Minor
- 10–30% of plasma cells on bone marrow biopsy
- Abnormal monoclonal band but less then above
- Lytic bone lesions
- Immune paresis

Answer continued overleaf

Other notes regarding the presentation of myeloma

- Patients may also present with symptoms suggestive of hypercalcaemia (bone pain, increased urinary frequency, confusion). Unless there are pathological fractures the alkaline phosphatase will be normal.
- The most serious complication of monoclonal protein production, particularly that resulting from excessive synthesis of Bence-Jones protein, is the development of potentially irreversible renal damage. Twenty five percent of patients with myeloma are uraemic at presentation and a further 25% show overt renal failure as the disease progresses. In over 95% of patients, renal failure is attributable to Bence-Jones protein and/ or hypercalcaemia.
- The hyperviscosity syndrome can occur because of agglutination of paraproteins in the microcirculation. This may lead to neurological disturbances such as confusion, fatigue and coma. There may be visual disturbances and retinal haemorrages.
- The hyperviscosity syndrome is particularly prominent with **Waldenstrom's macroglobulinaemia**. This is a lymphoplasmacytoid malignancy producing an IgM paraprotein, lymphadenopathy and splenomegaly.

3. Membranous glomerulosclerosis.

This is the commonest cause of nephrotic syndrome in adults and it is characterized by the presence of subepithelial immune deposits on the outer surface of the glomerular basement membrane. In children the commonest diagnosis is minimal change disease.

It may be associated in 20–25% of cases with:

Autoimmune disease
- Systemic lupus erythematosus
- Rheumatoid arthritis

Drugs
- Gold
- Penicillamine
- Captopril
- NSAIDS

Malignancy
- Bronchus, colon, stomach, prostate, breast
- Renal carcinoma
- Lymphoma

Infections
- Hepatitis B and C
- Syphilis
- Filariasis
- Leprosy
- Malaria

Miscellaneous
- Autoimmune thyroid disease
- Diabetes mellitus

The clinical course is variable and patients with an underlying cause usually respond to treatment. In patients with a normal creatinine 30% have complete remission.

3. Gilbert's syndrome.

The only abnormality is an elevated level of unconjugated bilirubin and the episode of jaundice was preceded by loss of appetite with reduced calorie intake.

Gilbert's syndrome encompasses a number of inherited metabolic abnormalities (presumed autosomal dominant in nature) which result in mildly elevated levels of unconjugated bilirubin. In many patients the primary defect is one of conjugation due to low levels of bilirubin glucuronidase. The elevated bilirubin level is usually insufficient to produce clinical jaundice. The diagnosis is usually made when calorie intake is reduced. This has the effect of raising serum levels of unconjugated bilirubin in the absence of haemolysis. On reducing calorie intake to less than 400 calories, unconjugated bilirubin levels double in normal patients and also those with Gilbert's disease. In the latter group, due to the higher starting value, clinical jaundice is often apparent.

A nicotinic acid provocation test may also be used to aid diagnosis. Intravenous nicotinic acid elevates the level of unconjugated bilirubin by at least 17 µmol/L and there is delayed clearance compared to normal controls. Liver biopsy is not essential for diagnosis; the histology is usually unremarkable but may show an increase in centrilobular lipofuscin. The long-term prognosis is excellent.

Other notes
- If this patient had been suffering from haemolytic anaemia he would also be expected to have an unconjugated hyperbilirubinaemia (bilirubin would not be detectable in the urine), he would be anaemic, the reticulcyte count might be raised, and a raised haptoglobulin level might be given.

Inherited defects in bilirubin metabolism				
Clinical syndrome	Conjugated/ unconjugated	Clinical presentation	Metabolic defect	Inheritance
Gilbert's	Unconjugated hyperbiliru-binaemia	Mild intermittent jaundice Normal hepatic biochemistry and hepatic histology Levels elevated with stress, fatigue, intercurrent illness	Low UDPGT1	Autosomal dominant (some variation in promotor gene defects and may be expressed as autosomal recessive
Crigler Najjar type 1	Unconjugated hyperbiliru-binaemia	Kernicterus in infancy	Absent UDPGT1	Autosomal recessive
Crigler Najjar type 2	Unconjugated hyperbiliru-binaemia	Survival into adult life with intermittent jaundice	Decreased UGPT1	Autosomal recessive
Dubin Johnson	Conjugated	Intermittent jaundice; black pigmented liver is a cardinal feature	Impaired transport protein	Autosomal recessive
Rotor	Conjugated	Intermittent jaundice	Molecular basis not determined	Autosomal recessive

3. Lewy body dementia.

- The presence of frank dementia and pyramidal signs indicate widespread disease such as diffuse Lewy body dementia, Alzheimer's disease or cerebrovascular disease causing multi-infarct dementia. In the latter there may be a short stepping gait which is upright and military (marche a petit pas); there may be a pseudobulbar palsy and emotional incontinence.
- Parkinsonian features may be apparent in any diffuse brain disease causing generalized cerebral damage. In addition to dementia, paralysis and other signs of widespread brain damage, an akinetic-rigid syndrome can occur.
- Increasing rigidity a resting tremor, micrographia and a festinant gait would all be typical features of idiopathic Parkinson's disease. Parkinson's disease can be considered to be a triad of tremor, rigidity and bradykinesia.
- Classically though, in such patients, mental function is preserved although it may deteriorate later in the disease and patients may become confused due to the toxic effects of dopaminergic drugs or concurrent illness.

A number of other degenerative diseases affecting the basal ganglia may produce a Parkinsonian syndrome and other associated features can indicate a 'Parkinson plus' type syndrome.

Diffuse brain diseases causing multifocal dementia in adults in which elements of parkinsonism may also occur:

Common
- Alzheimer's disease (including senile dementia)
- Diffuse Lewy body disease
- Multi-infarct dementia
- Amyloid angiopathy
- Head injury (e.g. boxers)
- Cerebral anoxia

Rare
- Pick's disease
- Creutzfeldt-Jacob disease
- Manganese poisoning
- Neurosyphilis
- Cystercercosis
- Communicating hydrocephalus

- In general, these conditions show little or no response to treatment with levodopa or dopamine agonists.
- A gaze palsy for voluntary and following eye movements, particularly when down-gaze is affected, with preserved vestibulo-ocular reflex eye movements, indicates progressive supranuclear palsy (Steele Richardson Olszewski syndrome).

- A cerebellar ataxia or cerebellar atrophy on CT scan, and orthostatic hypotension with other features of an autonomic neuropathy, point to multiple system atrophy (see 'Other Notes' below).
- Severe rigidity of a limb, with apraxia and myoclonus, suggests corticobasal degeneration.

Other notes

Multiple – system atrophy (MSA) is a neurodegenerative disease that leads to a Parkinson-plus phenotype and prominent autonomic changes. In addition to presenting with parkinsonism patients may also have autonomic symptoms: fatigue, weakness, orthostatic dizziness, decreased sweating, bladder dysfunction, erectile dysfunction, changes in bowel motility and sleep abnormalities. Four clinical syndromes have been included within the diagnosis of MSA:

1. Pure autonomic failure (the Shy-Drager syndrome)
2. Striatonigral degeneration with a predominance of parkinsonism
3. Olivopontocerebellar degeneration with a predominance of cerebellar dysfunction
4. A combination of these syndromes

5. Polyarteritis nodosa.

Polyarteritis nodosa is the most likely diagnosis. This is a condition characterized by a necrotizing vasculitis affecting the medium-sized muscular arteries. These arterioles often develop aneurysmal swellings. Sometimes they can be palpated as nodules along superficial arteries.

- Typically a patient is middle aged and males are more commonly affected. He will present with fever, weight loss and night sweats. He may have abdominal pain secondary to intestinal ischaemia.
- There is an increased incidence of presentation in patients with hepatitis B.
- There are no specific diagnostic features. Anti Neutrophil Cytoplasmic Antibodies (ANCA) are usually negative.
- Angiographic studies will reveal evidence of vasculitis in muscular arteries with aneurysmal formation.
- Treatment is with corticosteroids and cytotoxic drugs. Patients with concurrent hepatitis B should receive appropriate antiviral treatment, e.g. with lamivudine.
- The right median nerve palsy suggests a mononeuritis multiplex; this is a well-recognized manifestation of polyarteritis nodosa.

Other notes
- **Wegener's granulomatosis** is a granulomatous small/medium vasculitis affecting the upper respiratory tract, the lower respiratory tract and the kidneys. Eighty five percent of patients are antiproteinase 3 antibody positive (c– ANCA +).
- **Henoch-Schönlein purpura** is characterized by the association of arthritis, palpable purpura, gut symptoms, and glomerulonephritis which is an IgA nephropathy. Patients initially notice urticarial spots over the extensor surfaces of the arms and legs, particularly around the ankles, buttocks and elbows with sparing of the face and trunk. The purpuric lesions can coalesce and become necrotic. Two-thirds of patients have a large joint flitting arthritis. Abdominal symptoms include abdominal pain, melaena, haematemesis and obstruction due to intramural haematomas and intussusception. An upper respiratory tract infection is a common precipitant. The diagnosis is confirmed by the finding of positive immunoflourescence for IgA and C3 within vasculitic lesions and on kidney biopsy. Fifty percent of patients will have elevated serum IgA concentrations.
- **C1-esterase deficiency** is more likely to present with abdominal symptoms and an angioedematous rash.
- **Kawasaki's disease** is an acute febrile disease which classically affects the coronary arteries and occurs in infants and children under 5 years.

a) 4. Recurrent lymphoma with *Pneumocystis carinii* infection.

b) 2. Bronchoscopy with washings and transbronchial biopsy.

4. CT scan of abdomen.

5. Liver biopsy.

Hodgkin's disease (Thomas Hodgkin, 1832) is commoner overall in males, with two age peaks of 15–25 and 55–75 years of age. The disease is characterized by the presence of Reed-Sternberg cells.

- Four histological variants are described: (i) lymphocyte predominant (10–15%; overall, this variant has the best prognosis); (ii) mixed cellularity (20–40%); (iii) lymphocyte depleted (5–15%); (iv) nodular sclerosing (20–50%).
- Clinically, patients present with enlarged lymph nodes (usually in the neck or axilla) or a mediastinal mass on chest X-ray. Twenty five percent of patients have constitutional or B symptoms of pruritus, fever, alcohol-induced pain and >10% weight loss.
- Staging is according to the Ann Arbor classification.

Ann Arbor classification	
Stage I	A single lymph node or a single extralymphatic organ or site.
Stage II	Two or more lymph node regions or an extranodal site and lymph nodes, on the same side of the diaphragm.
Stage III	Nodes on both sides of the diaphragm, with or without splenic involvement
Stage IV	Diffuse involvement of one or more extralymphatic sites, with or without lymphadenopathy.

- Treatment, broadly, is mantle or inverted Y radiotherapy for stages I and II disease (unless bulky). Stage III and IV disease, along with bulky stage II disease, are treated with a type of combination chemotherapy using a minimum of four drugs, an example being the ABVD regimen (doxorubicin, bleomycin, vinblastine and dacarbazine).

Five-year survival without treatment is 10%; now it is 80–90% for all stages with treatment. Early stage, youth, the absence of B symptoms and good prognostic histology bode best.

The disease caused by *Pneumocystis carinii* is an extensive pneumonitis found almost exclusively in the immunosuppressed or immunodeficient host.

- Pathologically the disease is characterized by an extensive desquamative alveolitis. The organisms are clustered in the alveolar lumen. The 'foamy exudate' formerly described represents unstained clusters of cysts and alveolar cells with cytoplasmic vacuoles.
- Clinical features include marked tachypnoea, dry cough and fever. Hypoxia is often marked and precedes radiological change. The typical

X-ray shows diffuse, bilateral alveolar disease originating at the hilum and progressing peripherally.

- For a definitive diagnosis, *P. carinii* must be identified in lung tissue by fibre-optic bronchoscopy or open lung biopsy.
- Treatment is with either (i) trimethoprim-sulphamethoxazole (co-trimoxazole) or (ii) pentamidine isothionate. Untreated, the fatality rate approaches 100%, but is reduced to 25% with one of these agents. Up to 15% of patients who recover will have a second episode. Chemoprophylaxis for high-risk patients is with co-trimoxazole, which is dependable for only as long as the drug is taken.

a) 3. Primary hyperparathyroidism.

b) 3. Peptic ulceration.

c) 5. Measure parathyroid hormone levels.

In 80% of cases patients who present with **primary hyperparathyroidism** have a single adenoma; diffuse gland hyperplasia accounts for approximately 10% and multiple adenomas for 4% of cases. Investigations show hypercalcaemia, a low phosphate, a raised alkaline phosphatase, and a hyperchloraemic metabolic acidosis due to an associated distal (type I) renal tubular acidosis. The elevated blood urea may be explained by dehydration subsequent to polyuria induced by the hypercalcaemia.

These changes are typical of primary hyperparathyroidism and do not tend to occur in other causes of hypercalcaemia. The diagnosis is confirmed by finding an inappropriately high parathyroid hormone level for the serum calcium.

There is a well-recognized association between primary hyperparathyroidism and peptic ulceration, which explains the epigastric pain (note: a gastrointestinal bleed could also account for the elevated urea). Fifty percent of patients with primary hyperparathyroidism will develop renal stones. However, most patients with primary hyperparathyroidism are diagnosed on routine screening and are asymptomatic.

Clinical features of hypercalcaemia
- Abdominal pain
- Constipation
- Nausea and vomiting
- Renal colic
- Polydipsia
- Polyuria
- Peptic ulceration
- Pancreatitis
- Weakness
- Psychiatric changes
- Band keratopathy of the cornea
- Association with other tumours*

*Primary hyperparathyroidism, pituitary tumours, pancreatic tumours and adrenal cortical tumours – multiple endocrine neoplasia type I (MEN type I). Primary hyperparathyroidism, medullary carcinoma of the thyroid, phaeochromocytomas, carcinoid tumours (MEN type II) (and mucosal neuromas MEN IIb).

Other features of primary hyperparathyroidism
1. A hyperchloraemic metabolic acidosis (unlike other cases of hypercalcaemia)
2. Elevated 24-h urinary calcium excretion
3. Elevated urinary cAMP
4. Elevated urinary hydroxyproline excretion
5. Radiology: subperiosteal bone resorption, bone cysts, brown tumours and deformities
6. The hydrocortisone suppression test fails to suppress calcium levels in primary hyperparathyroidism but does so in other cases of hypercalcaemia.

Other notes
- A diagnosis of myeloma is made less likely if:
  - there is a normal full blood count
  - there is a normal ESR
  - the total protein count and albumin are normal (elevated protein and reduced albumin would be expected with immunoglobulin production)
  - the phosphate is likely to be in the normal range in myeloma
  - the alkaline phosphatase is usually normal unless there are healing fractures
  - deranged renal function would be more likely.
- A diagnosis of chronic renal failure is made less likely if there is:
  - a normal full blood count
  - low phosphate
  - a normal level of creatinine and urea.

a) 5. Chronic hepatitis B infection with high infectivity.

b) 3. Chronic active hepatitis on liver biopsy.

4. HBV DNA polymerase detected in the serum.

It is most likely that this patient acquired infection during childhood. The factors that determine whether a patient develops chronic hepatitis B infection or recovers fully are not known. After an acute infection 10% of patients develop one of three chronic syndromes: (i) chronic carrier HBs Ag positive, HBe Ag negative, but with normal histology; (ii) chronic persistent hepatitis, characterized by asymptomatic mild elevation transaminases, no piecemeal necrosis and no cirrohosis; (iii) chronic active hepatitis characterized by active inflammation, and hepatic necrosis which may progress to cirrhosis and is an important risk for the development of primary hepatocellular carcinoma.

Remember: During the first years of chronic infection, virus replication is high; patients are HBs Ag and HBe Ag positive but are e antibody negative and are highly infectious. Later, patients develop antibodies to first HBc Ag (IgM implies recent infection and IgG implies chronic infection), then HBe Ag and finally HBs Ag. After many years antibodies to HBs Ag and HBe Ag may be undetectable, although antibodies to the core protein (HBc Ag) remain detectable.

Indications for therapy include: infectivity, e.g. HBe Ag-positive patients, and evidence of progressive liver disease (chronic active hepatitis) and detectable HBV DNA polymerase in the serum. Decompensated cirrhosis is a contraindication. Treatment with antiviral agents, e.g. limivudine and possibly interferon, is useful even if the virus has become integrated into the host genome; improvement of the inflammatory liver disease will occur if viral replication is inhibited.

4. Vitamin K 1 mg IV.

- The most appropriate treatment would be to give a low dose of IV vitamin K.
- Rapid control of bleeding is not required providing the patient is stable.
- If too much vitamin K is given it will have a long-term effect on the vitamin K dependent clotting system and disrupt warfarin control for weeks.

Treatment for patients on warfarin therapy with an elevated INR

For major bleeding
- Stop warfarin
- Give vitamin K 5 mg slow IV.
- Give prothrombin concentrate (factors II, VII, IX, X) 50 units/kg
- If there is no concentrate available then FFP (15 mL/kg)

If the INR is >8 and there is no bleeding or minor bleeding
- Stop warfarin
- Give vitamin K either 0.5–1 mg IV or 5 mg po. Repeat the dose if the INR is too high

If the INR is 6.0–8.0
- Stop the warfarin and remeasure the INR when it is less then 5.0

---

1. Hypoglycaemia unawareness syndrome.

The results of the diabetic care and complication trial (DCCT) demonstrate that strict glycaemic control in patients with type 1 diabetes mellitus (DM) significantly reduces microvascular endpoints such as retinopathy, neuropathy and microalbuminduria.

Despite these reductions, patients experienced a three-fold increase in severe hypoglycaemia. Hypoglycaemia unawareness is associated with intensified insulin therapy. It can be resolved by avoiding hypoglycaemia for about 1 month.

Severe hypoglycaemia is often associated with an adrenergic response (pallor, tachycardia, sweating and anxiety). If untreated it can lead to CNS glucose deprivation, confusion, seizures and coma. These adrenergic responses are lost in the hypoglycaemia unawareness syndrome but return providing hypoglycaemia can be avoided for 4-6 weeks.

Note: this patient is not Addisonian. The low sodium is a common side-effect of carbamazepine treatment and is usually well tolerated.

Answer to question 154

4. Neuroleptic malignant syndrome.

This is a well-recognized idiosyncratic side-effect of antidopaminergic drugs such as phenothiazines and butyrophenones, which are used in the management of schizophrenia. The syndrome usually develops insidiously soon after treatment is initiated, and is characterized by hyperthermia, tachycardia, muscle rigidity, dysphagia and impaired consciousness. Creatinine kinase levels are elevated and reflect muscle damage. Death from respiratory failure is not uncommon; other complications include renal failure due to myoglobinuria, metabolic acidosis and cardiac failure. The increased muscle tone appears to be presynaptically mediated and recovery occurs when neuroleptic serum levels fall.

Management of the syndrome includes active cooling, rehydration, correction of metabolic acidosis, and ventilation when necessary. Intravenous dantrolene, which inhibits calcium efflux from muscle, and dopamine antagonists, e.g. bromocriptine, have been used with varying effect to reduce muscle tone.

a) 2. septic arthritis of the left knee.

Although this is unlikely, **septic arthritis** of the left knee must be excluded in view of the fever, very high CRP, new joint presentation and immunosupression due to steroid usage. All joints that are involved in an inflammatory or degenerative process are at increased risk of becoming infected.

b) 2. Rheumatoid arthritis.

Rheumatoid arthritis is the most likely diagnosis. This is a symmetrical, deforming, peripheral arthropathy, (affecting all synovial joints) with a peak onset of 40 years of age, although it can occur earlier. The ratio for female to male is 3:1. It typically presents with swollen, painful and stiff hands and feet, especially in the morning. This gradually gets worse and larger joints are involved. There is inflammation of the synovium with destruction of cartilage, loss of joint space, tendon ruptures and subsequent destruction of the joint. Rheumatoid factor is positive in 75% but is not specific. Anticyclical citrillinated peptide antibody is highly specific with a sensitivity approaching 70%.

Extra-articular manifestations tend to be more severe with high titres of antirheumatoid factor. Extra-articular manifestations include nodules, anaemia, lymphadenopathy, pleurisy, pleural effusions (commoner in males), pericarditis, episcleritis, scleritis, keratoconjunctivitis, osteoporosis, secondary amyloidosis, vasculitis and in 1% Felty's syndrome (splenomegaly, leucopenia, lymphadenopathy, skin ulcers, anaemia and thrombocytopenia).

c) 5. Aspiration of synovial fluid from left knee for microscopy and culture.
8. Blood cultures.

Microscopy and culture of blood and synovial fluid are required to exclude infection.

An isotope bone scan will not be helpful in this case as there is obvious joint involvement. It is useful in patients with joint pains and stiffness with no acute inflammatory response or obvious joint deformity. This will show early synovitis where X-rays are normal.

Note: gout is extremely rare in premenopausal women.

3. Osteomalacia.

This is suggested by:

- A history of fatigue, and there is a suggestion of proximal muscle weakness (increased immobility and difficulty getting out of the chair)
- A hypophosphataemia with a low plasma calcium concentration; her ALP is raised and given her symptoms, this is likely to be bony in origin
- Vitamin D deficiency due to inadequate nutritional intake and reduced exposure to sunlight, which is more common in the immigrant Asian population; classically, there is low serum calcium and low phosphate with an elevated alkaline phosphatase, and increased urinary phosphate excretion due to secondary hyperparathyroidism (there may be a secondary mild hyperchloraemic acidosis).

Osteomalacia and rickets are characterized by defective mineralization of bone and cartilage leading to an accumulation of unmineralized bone matrix called osteoid. Rickets occurs before there has been fusion of the epiphyses in children.

- The most common causes of osteomalacia are due to defects in vitamin D metabolism, or less commonly, to defects in renal handling of phosphate.
- Characteristic symptoms are generalized bone pain and tenderness associated with weakness of the proximal muscles. The bone pain is poorly localized and often made worse with walking.
- The radiological hallmark of active osteomalacia is the Looser's zone. This is a ribbon-like area of defective mineralization, which may be found in almost any bone but is seen particularly in the long bones, pelvis, ribs, and also around the scapulae. The vertebral bodies are often uniformly biconcave, and produce an appearance likened to a 'fish spine'.
- In patients with osteomalacia and hypocalcaemia the radiological features of secondary hyperparathyroidism can appear with subperiosteal bone resorption, which affects the phalanges, the pubic symphysis, and the outer ends of the clavicles.

Summary of causes of osteomalacia
1. Abnormal vitamin D metabolism
Reduced availability

- Nutrition
- Inadequate exposure to sunlight
- Malabsorption states – (gastrectomy, coeliac disease, Crohn's disease, pancreatic insufficiency, hepatobiliary disease)

Defective metabolism

- Hepatobiliary disease
- Chronic renal failure
- Anticonvulsant drugs
- Vitamin D dependent rickets type I and II*
- Malignancy
- X-linked hypophosphataemia

2. Renal phosphate loss

- X-linked hypophosphataemia#
- Fanconi syndromes, type II renal tubular acidosis
- Malignancies

3. Others

- Aluminium toxicity – (deposited in bone and impairs mineralization)
- Antacid abuse, malabsorption

* *Vitamin D dependent rickets types I and II*

- Type I is an autosomal recessive condition where there is a defect in 1Alpha hydroxylase activity. Rickets presents before 3 years of age. Vitamin D levels are undetectable.
- Type II is an X-linked dominant condition where there is a receptor defect. Alopecia is common.

X-linked hypophosphataemic rickets (vitamin D resistant rickets)
The inheritance is X-linked dominant in the majority of cases. It is fully expressed in the homozygous state in males and the expression in females is variable. A low serum phosphate level is characteristic and children have severe rickets and stunted growth.

Other notes
Causes of hypocalcaemia and hyperphosphataemia

- Primary hypoparathyroidism
- Renal failure
- Pseudohypoparathyroidism

Other conditions causing hypocalcaemia

- Magnesium deficiency (sometimes seen with cytotoxic drugs)
- Renal tubular disorders
- Acute pancreatitis
- Rhabdomyolysis

1. Tighter insulin control.

The clearest evidence comes from the DCCT (Diabetes Control and Complications Trial) that reducing HbAIC levels and tight glycaemic control results in decreased microvascular endpoints by 30%.

Among white patients in the UK with type I diabetes of 15–30 years duration, fewer then 20% will have established nephropathy.

In patients with type II diabetes, nephropathy is closely associated with large vessel disease. Lipid-lowering treatment, aspirin, beta blockers, angiotension-converting enzyme inhibitors and insulin treatment after myocardial infarction have all had beneficial effects on cardiovascular mortality, and therefore, more patients are surviving to endstage renal failure.

Microalbuminuria (3–300 mg/24 h) is the first marker of diabetic nephropathy and a valuable marker of risk in type II diabetes. It also correlates strongly with diabetic control.

The albumin to creatinine ratio is simpler to collect and has a good correlation with the timed albumin excretion.

All patients with negative protein on conventional urinalysis are annually screened for microalbuminuria. A urinary albumin:creatinine ratio of >2.5 mg/mmol in men and >3.5 mg/mol in women should trigger a timed urine collection and consideration of further treatment.

Management of nephropathy centres on aggressive antihypertensive control (with a target blood pressure of 130/80 mmHg) and inhibition of the renin angiotension system. (micropuncture studies show that they reduce intraglomerular pressure over and above the reduction in systemic blood pressure).

As discussed:
- ACEIs have been shown to have an advantage over previous anti-hypertensive agents.
- Angiotensin II antagonists are a more recent addition and have been shown to have equivalent effects on reducing progression from microalbuminuria to renal failure.

3. Posterior myocardial infarction.

The main ECG abnormalities are dominant R-waves in lead V1 and non-specific ST segment flattening in leads I and VL. The dominant R-waves in lead V1 might indicate right ventricular hypertrophy, but other features would also be expected, such as right axis deviation and T-wave inversion in the anterior chest leads (V1–V3).

A posterior myocardial infarction can be detected on the 12 lead ECG because it causes a dominant R-wave in lead V1. There may also be ischaemic ST segment depression in the anterior leads (V2–V4) – the mirror and inverted image of the pattern of changes seen in an anterior myocardial infarction.

Causes of a dominant R-wave in lead V1
Normal variant
Right bundle branch block
Right ventricular hypertrophy
Posterior myocardial infarction
Wolff-Parkinson-White syndrome
Dextrocardia, Duchenne muscular dystrophy

a) 5. Systemic lupus erythematosus.

b) 3. Anti-double stranded DNA titres.

This patient has many typical features of systemic lupus erythematosus (SLE), In addition she has evidence of active renal disease – her urine is positive for protein and blood and there are granular casts in the urinary sediment and her protein is in the nephrotic range. A renal biopsy would ascertain what class of lupus nephritis she has and this is important to plan management.

Systemic lupus erythematosus is an autoimmune multi-system disease, which typically affects females during childbearing age. It is more common amongst black females in the UK. Autoantibodies to DNA, ENA and other nuclear and cell surface antigens characterize it serologically.

- Positivity to antinuclear antibody is found in >99% of patients with SLE. Different staining patterns correspond to different antibody binding – the homogenous pattern corresponds to binding of ds DNA and/or histones. Speckled or nucleolar patterns can also occur. ANA negative patients genererally have antibodies to the antigens Ro and/or La and tend to have less renal disease.
- Anti-ds DNA antibodies are found in 40–90% of patients.
- Antibodies to extractable nuclear antigens (Ro, La, Sm, RNP) can be found in a third of patients. Antibodies to La are associated with Sjögren's syndrome.
- Antibodies to RNP are associated with undifferentiated autoimmune rheumatic disease. Anti-sm antibodies are highly specific for SLE but do not have a disease association.
- Pharmacological treatment of patients depends on their specific manifestations. Generally, patients with mild/moderate disease are treated with combinations of NSAIDS, antimalarials and oral corticosteroids. More powerful immunosuppressive agents are required (azathioprine and cyclophosphamide) for more severe manifestations and severe renal disease. Arterial and venous thromboses are treated conventionally.
- The best serological markers of disease activity are the erythrocyte sedimentation rate, reduced complement levels and high anti-ds DNA titres

The majority of patients will develop abnormalities of their urine or renal function in the course of their disease. Proteinuria dominates the clinical presentation. About one-quarter of patients will show a nephrotic syndrome in the course of their disease. Over half will have reduced renal function, but they rarely present with acute renal failure. Renal artery thrombosis can occur often in the presence of the antiphospholipid antibody and can be associated with acute deterioration in renal function.

The histology of lupus nephritis is divided into six types and this helps to plan therapy and prognosis.

SLE is diagnosed if four or more of the following eleven features are present together or serially.

Malar rash
A fixed erythematous, flat or raised rash
A classical butterfly rash found over the bridge of the nose and malar bones is present in two-thirds of patients

Discoid rash
Present in 15% of patients
Erythematous raised patches with adherent keratotic scaling and follicular plugging; atrophic scarring may occur

Photosensitivity
Exposure to UV light causes the rash, which accounts for its distribution over areas exposed to the sun

Oral ulceration
Includes oral and nasopharyngeal ulceration
Anorexia and abdominal pain can also occur
Mucosal ulcers can become deep and infected with *Candida*

Arthritis
A non-erosive arthritis involving two or more peripheral joints, characterized by tenderness, swelling or effusion
Musculoskeletal features affect more than 90% of patients

Serositis
Pleuritic **or** pericarditis documented by ECG or rub, or evidence of a pericardial effusion
Pulmonary disease occurs in 40% of patients; common manifestations are pleurisy or small pleural effusions
Parenchymal involvement is rare
Pericarditis is more common then myocarditis and patients can also develop an endocarditis (Libman-Sachs endocarditis)

Renal
Proteinuria >0.5 g/24 h or 3+ persistently **or** Cellular casts

Neurological
Seizures or psychosis without evidence of another cause
Almost any neurological abnormality can be present

Haematogical
Haemolytic anaemia **or**
Leucopenia <4.0 × 10^9/L on two or more separate occasions **or**
Lymphopenia <1.5 × 10^9/L on two or more occasions **or**
Thrombocytopenia <100 × 10^9/L
A normochromic haemolytic anaemia is present in 70% of patients and there is also commonly a Coombs' positive haemolytic anaemia

Immunological
Raised anti- ds DNA antibody binding **or** Anti Sm antibody **or**
Positive finding of antiphospholipid antibodies based on:
1. An abnormal level of serum IgG or IgM anticardiolipin antibodies
2. A positive test for the lupus anticoagulant
3. A false positive serological test for syphilis, present for at least 6 months

Anti-nuclear antibody in raised titre
An abnormal titre of ANA, in the absence of a history of the 'drug-induced lupus syndrome'

1. Serum transferrin and ferritin concentrations.

The underlying disorder in this patient was found to be haemachromatosis. See the answer to question 31 for a clinical description of haemachromatosis.

If all the above investigations are negative then patients are given the diagnosis of idiopathic hypogonadotrophic hypogonadism but haemachromatosis should always be excluded. Some of these patients are found to have Kallman's syndrome (described in the answer to question 27).

3. Commence a statin.

In patients with diabetes, premature atherosclerotic disease is the main cause of a reduced life expectancy. Hyperglycaemia is known to be the major risk factor for microvascular complications; cigarette smoking, hypertension and dyslipidaemia are potent risk factors for macrovascular disease in patients with diabetes. Diabetes is also associated with an increase in the amount of small dense LDL particles, which are highly atherogenic.

Many of the clinical trials involving lipid lowering drugs as secondary preventative agents, such as the 4S and CARE trials, show a significant reduction in recurrent events. Some of the seminal primary prevention trials, such as the west of Scotland study and the AFCAPS/TexcCAPS study did not have enough patients to enable subgroup analysis.

Pooled analyses of some of these trials have also shown benefit in risk reduction in patients with other cardiac risk factors.

Other notes
- The role of fibrate therapy in type II diabetes has been shown to be effective in patients with secondary risk factors for atheroscelerotic disease but primary prevention trials have been performed only with small numbers.
- The Heart Protection study randomized over 20,000 patients aged 40–80 years, including 6000 with diabetes, to treatment with placebo or simvastatin 40 mg for 5.5 years. Overall the risk of acute myocardial infarction and stroke was reduced by a third. The HPS also found that vitamin C, vitamin E and beta-carotene were not associated with any benefit or major outcome.
- The current recommendation for primary prevention in patients is that a statin should be considered for patients with total serum cholesterol of 5 mmol/L or greater and a coronary heart disease risk of 30% or greater over 10 years. This risk can be calculated from risk prediction charts, e.g. the joint British societies' charts, published in the British National Formulary.

Answer to question 162

1. Pituitary microadenoma.

Prolactinomas are the commonest functioning pituitary tumours. (They are the commonest pituitary tumours occurring in multiple endocrine neoplasia type 1 (MEN type 1 = pituitary and parathyroid adenomas and pancreatic endocrine tumours).)

The main clinical features of hyperprolactinaemia secondary to micro/macro adenomas are:
- Galactorrhoea (90% in females and 10% males)
- Disturbed gonadal function:
  - females: menstrual disturbance – oligomenorrhoea, amenorrhoea or with infertility or reduced libido
  - males: loss of libido and erectile dysfunction; infertility and gynaecomastia are uncommon
- Mass effects: due to macroadenomas only – headaches and visual field defects, hypopituitarism, invasion of the cavernous sinus leading to cranial nerve palsies.

High prolactin levels may be seen in a variety of physiological and pathological conditions, see 'Causes of Hyperprolactinaemia' below. A prolactin concentration greater then 3000 mU/L, however, is highly likely to indicate a prolactinoma. This can either be a micro (<10 mm) or macro (>10 mm) adenoma. A serum prolactin concentration greater then 6000 mU/L is diagnostic of a macroprolactinoma.
- The dopamine antagonist test is sometimes used to differentiate between idiopathic hyperprolactaemia and an undetectable microprolactinoma. The secretion and release of prolactin is inhibited by dopamine. Any process that disrupts dopamine secretion or interferes with dopamine to the portal vessels can cause hyperprolactinaemia. Metoclopramide antagonises lactrotroph dopamine receptors leading to elevated prolactin levels.
- If metoclopramide is given intravenously to a normal patient or a patient with an elevated prolactin level not due to a prolactinoma, one would expect a 2-fold rise in the prolactin level, with no change in TSH. Prolactinomas will display a blunted prolactin response and an exaggerated TSH response.

The goal of treatment is to restore gonadal function and in the case of macroprolactinomas, to reduce tumour size (microprolactinomas very rarely expand in size).
- The two dopamine antagonists used are bromocriptine and cabergoline. D2 receptor stimulation leads to inhibition of prolactin secretion and hopefully tumour shrinkage. Cabergoline, which is longer acting, seems to be better tolerated then bromocriptine.

- Surgery is only indicated for patients who are intolerant or resistant to dopamine agonist treatment. The cure rate for macroprolactinomas is less then 50% and therefore conservative management is the primary treatment (providing there is no evidence of compression e.g.visual disturbance). About 75% of micro and macro adenomas respond to treatment.

Causes of hyperprolactinaemia

Physiological causes

- Pregnancy
- Exercise
- Post prandial
- Stimulation of chest wall (breastfeeding)

Pathological causes

- Physical/psychological stress
- Drugs: metoclopramide, phenothiazines, antidepressants – risperidone, monoamine oxidase inhibitors
- Pituitary tumours
- Pituitary gland infiltration
- Acromegaly
- Chronic renal failure
- Hypothyroidism.

Answer to question 163

a) 4. Adrenaline 1/1000 solution 0.5 mL IM.

b) 2. Measure serum mast cell tryptase.

Anaphylaxis describes a severe systemic allergic response and respiratory difficulty and/or hypotension is invariably present. In addition there are likely to be a number of other clinical features that are variably present (see the following box).

Anaphylaxis is, typically, a hypersensitivity reaction leading to sudden activation of mast cells and basophils mediated by immunoglobulin E. Cardiovascular collapse is caused by vasodilatation and loss of plasma from the blood compartment. Respiratory difficulty may be due to laryngeal oedema or asthma. Insect stings, drugs or contrast media, and some foods are the most common causes. In each case a thorough history and examination should be performed. Mast cell tryptase is a non-specific indicator of mast cell activation that can be raised in anaphylactic reactions and provides further evidence that an anaphylactic reaction has taken place.

Typical clinical features of an Anaphylactic Reaction

One or more features on the left are invariably present in association with a combination of features on the right.

Laryngeal oedema	Colour change: flushed or pale
Asthma	Erythema
Fainting and lightheadedness	Pruritis (generalized)
Cardiovascular collapse	Urticaria
Loss of consciousness	Angioedema
	Rhinitis
	Conjunctivitis
	Itching of palate or external auditory meatus
	Nausea, vomiting, abdominal pain
	Palpitations

Any of the features in the box can have a multitude of causes which may be misinterpreted as an 'allergic' reaction. Symptoms or clinical signs suggestive of features such as urticaria or angioedema may be classified and treated as 'anaphylactic' reactions when there has been no evidence of life-threatening features.

Anaphylactic reactions vary in severity and progress may be rapid, slow, or (unusually) biphasic.

Treatment

With evidence of severe features, prompt treatment is life saving.
Anaphylaxis should be considered:

- When there is a compatible history of severe allergic type reaction with respiratory difficulty and/or hypotension, especially when typical skin changes are present (urticaria and/or angioedema)

- If the patient is assessed and there is STRIDOR, WHEEZE and clinical signs of SHOCK:
  - adrenaline should be administered 0.5 mL 1/1000 solution (500 mcg) IM which may be repeated after 5 min.

Other treatments
- Antihistamine (chlorpheniramine) 10–20 mg IM/or slow IV

In addition:
- Hydrocortisone 100–500 mg IM/or slowly IV: for all severe or recurrent reactions and patients with asthma.
- If clinical manifestations of shock do not respond to drug treatment give 1–2 L IV fluid.

Other notes
- An inhaled beta 2-agonist such as salbutamol may be used as an adjunctive measure if bronchospasm is severe and does not respond rapidly to other treatment.
- If profound shock is judged to be immediately life-threatening, give CPR/ALS if necessary. Consider slow IV adrenaline (epinephrine) 1:10,000 solution. This is hazardous and is recommended only for an experienced practitioner who can also obtain IV access without delay. Note the different strength of adrenaline (epinephrine) that may be required for IV use.
- If adults are treated with an Epipen, 300 µg will usually be sufficient. A second dose may be required.
- Half doses of adrenaline (epinephrine) may be safer for patients on amitriptyline, imipramine, or beta blocker.
- A crystalloid may be safer than a colloid.

Answer to question 164

a) 2. Reversible obstructive airways disease.

Presumably this is an infective exacerbation of asthma in this case.

b) 3. Tracheal stricture.

The tracheal stricture is due to extrathoracic tracheal obstruction. Note that the diagram below represents a normal flow-volume loop.

The first flow-volume loop in the question is typical of severe obstructive airways disease, most commonly asthma or severe obstructive pulmonary disease. Maximal expiratory flow rates during the final part of expiration are largely effort independent and therefore vary directly with the elastic recoil of the lung and inversely with the airway resistance upstream of the equal pressure point. The normal expiratory limb in the second loop confirms that this must be reversible airways obstruction, i.e. asthma. The inspiratory limb of the second flow loop is abnormal. The MIF_{50} is the inspiratory flow rate at 50% of the vital capacity and, in this instance, is approximately half that expected. The midportion of the maximal inspiratory curve is flattened. This confirms an extrathoracic tracheal obstruction which must be variable as the expiratory limb is unaffected. In the clinical context, this is likely to be a consequence of long-term intubation, with development of a tracheal stricture – this patient should have been managed with a tracheostomy.

- Other causes of extrathoracic tracheal obstruction include vocal cord palsies, malignancy, and infective and inflammatory conditions, including Wegener's granulomatosis, relapsing polychondritis and syphilis.
- The other important pattern of flow-volume loop is that of a fixed intrathoracic tracheal obstruction, e.g. due to hilar malignancy, and in this instance, both the inspiratory and expiratory limbs will be flattened.

Flow volume loops measure the expiratory and inspiratory flow of air (L/s) against actual volume exhaled or inhaled.

- The (upper) expiratory curve starts with the patient at a maximum/forced inhalation (TLC) and ends at total forced exhalation (RV).
  The expiratory limb peaks rapidly (equivalent to the PEF obtained with a peak flow meter) maximum expiratory flow then declines progressively as volume is expired. In young healthy subjects the descending limb of the expiratory curve is roughly linear, whilst in older patients the expiratory flow decreases more rapidly at lower lung volumes so the curve has a more concave appearance. In patients with diffuse airways disease or narrowing such as in COPD or asthma this appearance is more marked.
- The (lower) maximum inspiratory flow-volume curve is more symmetrical – in patients with diffuse airway narrowing inspiratory flow is reduced, but little change in shape.

In patients with a restrictive ventilatory defect such as caused by pulmonary fibrosis the volume displaced will be reduced but flow rates are proportionally less affected. Localized narrowing of the proximal airways therefore also produce a characteristic pattern:

- Extrathoracic narrowing such as that occurring with tracheal stenosis has a relatively greater effect on inspiratory rather than expiratory flow. While it does affect the expiratory flow this only tends to occurs at higher lung volumes causing a flattening of the expiratory flow curve.
- Narrowing within the thorax caused for example by a hilar malignancy a similar plateau is seen but the inspiratory limb is proportionately less affected.

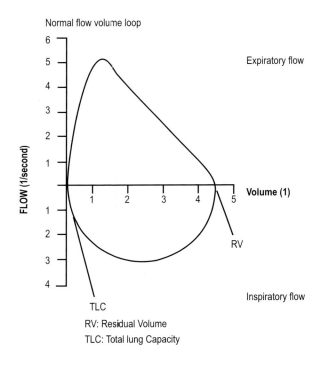

Normal flow volume loop

RV: Residual Volume
TLC: Total lung Capacity

Normal values

HAEMATOLOGY

Haemoglobin

Male	13.5–17.7 g/dL
Female	11.5–16.5 g/dL

Mean corpuscular haemoglobin (MCH)   27–32 pg
Mean corpuscular haemoglobin concentration (MCHC)   32–36 g/dL
Mean corpuscular volume (MCV)   80–96 fL

Packed cell volume (PCV)

Male	0.40–0.54 L/L
Female	0.37–0.47 L/L

White blood count (WBC)	$4–11 \times 10^9$/L
Basophil granulocytes	$<0.01–0.1 \times 10^9$/L
Eosinophil granulocytes	$0.04–0.4 \times 10^9$/L
Lymphocytes	$1.5–4.0 \times 10^9$/L
Monocytes	$0.2–0.8 \times 10^9$/L
Neutrophil granulocyes	$2.0–7.5 \times 10^9$/L

Total blood volume   60–80 mL/kg
Plasma volume   40–50 mL/kg
Platelet count $150–400 \times 10^9$/L
Serum B_{12} 160–925 ng/L (150–675 pmol/L)
Serum folate   2.9–18 µg/L (3.6–63 nmol/L)
Red cell folate   149–640 µg/L

Red cell mass

Male	25–35 mL/kg
Female	20–30 mL/kg

Reticulocyte count   0.5–2.5% of red cells ($50–100 \times 10^9$/L)
Erythrocyte sedimentation rate (ESR)   <20 mm in 1 hour
Plasma viscosity   1.5–1.72 mPa.s

Coagulation

Bleeding time (Ivy method)   3–9 min
Activated partial thromboplastin time (APTT)   23–31 s
Prothrombin time   12–16 s
   International Normalized Ratio (INR)   1.0–1.3
D-dimer   <500 ng/mL

Biochemistry (serum/plasma)

Alanine aminotransferase (ALT)   5–40 U/L
Albumin   35–50 g/L
Alkaline phosphatase   39–117 U/L
Amylase   25–125 U/L
Angiotensin-converting enzyme   10–70 U/L
α_1-antitrypsin   1.1–2.1 g/L
Aspartate aminotransferase (AST)   12–40 U/L
Bicarbonate   22–30 mmol/L
Bilirubin   <17 µmol/L (0.3–1.5 mg/dL)

Caeruloplasmin   0.20–0.61/L
Calcium   2.20–2.67 mmol/L (8.5–10.5 mg/dL)
Chloride   98–106 mmol/L
Complement
  C3   0.75–1.65 g/L
  C4   0.20–0.60 g/L
Copper   11–20 μmol/L (100–200 mg/dL)
C-reactive protein   <10 mg/L
Creatinine   79–118 μmol/L (0.6–1.5 mg/dL)
Creatine kinase (CPK)
  Female   24–170 U/L
  Male   24–195 U/L
  CK-MB fraction   <25 U/L (<60% of total activity)
Ferritin
  Female   6–110 μg/L
  Male   20–260 μg/L
  Post menopausal   12–230 μg/L
α-fetoprotein   <10 k U/L
Glucose (fasting)   4.5–5.6 mmol/L (70–110 mg/dL)
Fructosamine   up to 285 μmol/L
γ-glutamyl transpeptidase (γ-GT)
  Male   11–58 U/L
  Female   7–32 U/L
Glycosylated (glycated) haemoglobin (HbA$_{1c}$)   3.7–5.1%
Hydroxybutyric dehydrogenase (HBD)   72–182 U/L
Immunoglobulins (11 years and over)
  IgA   0.8–4 g/L
  IgG   5.5–16.5 g/L
  IgM   0.4–2.0 g/L
Iron   13–32 μmol/L (50–150 μg/dL)
Iron binding capacity (total) (TIBC)   42–80 μmol/L (250–410 μg/dL)
Lactate dehydrogenase   240–480 U/L
Magnesium   0.7–1.1 mmol/L
β$_2$-microglobulin   1.0–3.0 mg/L
Osmolality   275–295 mOsm/kg
Phosphate   0.8–1.5 mmol/L
Potassium   3.5–5.0 mmol/L
Prostate-specific antigen (PSA) up to 4.0 μg/L
Protein (total)   62–77 g/L
Sodium   135–146 mmol/L
Urate   0.18–0.42 mmol/L (3.0–7.0 mg/dL)
Urea   2.5–6.7 mmol/L (8–25 mg/dL)
Vitamin A   0.5–2.01 μmol/L
Vitamin D
  25-hydroxy   37–200 nmol/L (0.15–0.80 ng/L)
  1,25-dihydroxy   60–108 pmol/L (0.24–0.45 pg/L)
Zinc   11–24 μmol/L

Normal values

Lipids and lipoproteins

Cholesterol   3.5–6.5 mmol/L (ideal <5.2 mmol/L)
HDL cholesterol
Male	0.8–1.8 mmol/L
Female	1.0–2.3 mmol/L

LDL cholesterol   <4.0 mmol/L
Lipids (total)   4.0–10.0 g/L
Lipoproteins
VLDL	0.128–0.645 mmol/L
LDL	1.55–4.4 mmol/L
HDL	
Male	0.70–2.1 mmol/L
Female	0.50–1.70 mmol/L

Phospholipid   2.9–5.2 mmol/L
Triglycerides
Male	0.70–2.1 mmol/L
Female	0.50–1.70 mmol/L

Blood gases (arterial)

$P_a CO_2$ 4.8–6.1 kPa (36–46 mmHg)
$P_a O_2$ 10–13.3 kPa (75–100 mmHg)
[H+]   35–45 nmol/L
pH   7.35–7.45
Bicarbonate   22–26 mmol/L

Urine values

Calcium   7.5 mmol daily or less (<300 mg daily)
Copper   0.2–1.0 µmol daily
Creatinine   0.13–0.22 mmol per kilogram body weight, daily
5-hydroxyindole acetic acid (5HIAA) <75 µmol daily; amounts lower in females than males
Protein (quantitative)   <0.15 g per 24 hours
Sodium   60–80 mmol per 24 hours

Urine

Urine osmolality	60–1500 mOsmKg
Urine pH	4.6–8.0

Hormone levels

TSH	0.3–6 mU/L
fT4	9–22 pmol/L

Cerebrospinal fluid values

Opening pressure	7–18 cm/CSF
Protein	0.15–0.45 g/L
Glucose	2.8–4.2 mmol/L, CSF: blood glucose ratio >50%
Cell count	0.5 mm^3 all lymphocytes

Misc
ASOT   <200 iu/L

Haematology
Fibrinogen   2–4 g/dL
Thrombin Time   15–19 sec

Cardiology normal values

	Mean (mmHg)	Range (mmHg)
R.A.	4	0–8
R.V.		
systolic	25	15–30
end diastolic	4	0–8
P.A.P.		
systolic	25	15–30
diastolic	10	5–15
mean	15	10–20
P.A.W.P.	10	5–14
L.V.		
systolic	120	90–140
end diastolic	7	4–12
Aorta		
systolic	120	90–140
diastolic	70	60–90
mean	85	70–105

Index

Index

Note: Numbers refer to questions not pages.

Index

Index